Liver Cleanse
Reset and Detox

Moneva Amanda

ISBN: 978-1-63750-310-2

Table of Contents

Preface

"I've been looking forward to this book...It's exactly what I need to jump start my sluggish metabolism and give me the energy I need to lose those last few pounds I want to rid myself of!" -Prisca Sidoti, New York.

The Liver is a vital part of our body that performs countless important functions. It manufactures proteins, cleans the blood, filters the bile, breaks down toxins and plays a central role in cholesterol metabolism. Because of its importance, it is susceptible to damage from alcohol, tobacco, drugs, certain foods and a variety of other factors in our modern-day lifestyle. This can lead to a wide variety of uncomfortable symptoms like fatigue, bloating, discomfort, indigestion and more.

What if there was a simple way to cleanse and detoxify your liver and restore its natural ability to perform at optimal levels? *Would you be interested?*

Cleanse your liver and flush out toxins fast and easy with

this groundbreaking Book. With simple diet changes and special great insights, this fast-paced plan eliminates alcohol, caffeine, sugar, nicotine and other common toxins that can damage your liver. By flushing these substances out of your body, this program allows your liver to heal and rejuvenate itself. This is the most powerful detoxification system in the world, proven in scientific studies to:

- Remove up to 95% of toxins (including a wide variety of heavy metals) from your body
- Increase the efficiency of your liver by 50%,
- Reduce or even eliminate symptoms associated with stress and anxiety
- Improve your immune function and protect against chronic disease
- Decrease fat accumulation in the liver and improve insulin resistance
- Reduce or even eliminate constipation,
- Flush out stored water from your body
- Purge unwanted cholesterol and triglycerides
- Regain a healthy balance of electrolytes and flush out excess fluid

Do you want to live o 100 years?

Detoxifying your body is the best way to boost your energy levels, lose weight, get healthy, and make you feel years younger. It's easy to do. However, most people don't have the time or patience to do it properly. That's where this book comes in. It'll show you exactly what you need to do… and… it'll do it easily and quickly so you can start reaping the amazing health benefits of a liver detox.

Why not dive straight into the book, and thank me later…

Introduction

The body, whether we like to admit it or not, is deteriorating at a much faster pace because of the increasing level of toxins in our environment. Indeed, there is now technology to ease the symptoms that people are experiencing from the everyday poisons that enter our organs, but these medications and short-term remedies are just temporary.

If we continue to live our lives the same way by eating processed foods and consuming alcohol or drugs, we will certainly have the same signs and symptoms. And what's even worse is that these drugs which are taken to alleviate the pain also pose an unhealthy threat to your system once you take them continuously.

The liver is the first defense against all the harmful toxins that enter the body. However, because of the overload of harmful toxins that people continuously take in, it might begin to deteriorate and fail. Therefore, what can we do to help the liver?

We should concentrate on a diet plan that helps to cleanse and detoxify the liver. This is necessary because, at every point, it is important to revitalize the liver and remove every trace of harmful toxins in it. After this, we should begin to cultivate the conscious effort of living healthily, which will obviously start from the home.

This book can help you reset your liver and give it a whole new beginning. It contains the synopsis of a cleansing and detox plan, including specific actions on how to cleanse and detoxify this organ.

You should note that people who currently have a medical issue such as diabetes or a pre-existing liver problem should consult their general practitioner before undergoing any kind of at-home treatment.

There is no better time than now to save yourself from cancer of the liver before it's too late.

Chapter 1

The Roles and Functions of the Liver

The multiple functions of the liver can be divided into two general functions:

- To produce the essential molecules for the body (nutrition).

- To rid your body of dangerous toxins and pathogens (removal and defense).

Do you know?

The numerous activities of the liver include producing heat and raising the body temperature. The liver is generally 102.2° to 105.8°F i.e. it is hotter than other bodies. When we eat too much, the heat produced by the liver is increased, and this is communicated to other organs in the body. This explains why we feel warm whenever we are eating a big meal.

An Organ with Multiple Functions

The liver performs more than 500 functions. No other organ performs these varieties of tasks. Amazingly, the liver performs many of these tasks simultaneously.

Do you know?

The significance of the liver is revealed in its etymology. In British, the word liver is close to the word "live". The same in German, where liver (Leber) and life (Leben) are quite close.

Storage of Blood sugar and Rules of Glycemia

The energetic fuel that the cells use is a sugar known as glucose. To compensate for the inconsistent way to get sugar from food due to the time intervals between foods, the liver transforms sugar into glycogen. The liver then stores it in its tissues as a reserve, to be supplied to the blood as needed. Every time the blood sugar levels (glycemia) fall the liver changes this glycogen back to glucose, after which it is discharged into the blood to keep up with the right glycemia level for the effective functioning of the body.

If we didn't have a liver, we'd be constantly losing energy. When the foods we eat do not generate enough carbohydrates to be transformed into glycogen, the liver will produce them from fats or proteins.

On the contrary, whenever we are ingesting too many carbohydrates and the liver's glycogen reserves are full, extra sugar is stored in the liver using fat.

This fat overload weakens the liver and hinders it from functioning properly.

Storage of Nutrition and Regulations of Levels

Along with blood sugar, the liver stores all types of other nutritional requirements:

- Nutritional vitamins A and D.
- Various B vitamins, such as vitamin B12, a deficiency that can cause pernicious anemia.
- Iron, copper, etc.

When the blood level of these nutrients drops, the liver produces more into the blood to take it back again to normal. When the liver does not have these nutrients, deficiency ailments appear.

Production of Proteins

The protein entering the liver through the vein is changed there into different proteins that are helpful to your body. They include:

- **Albumin**: This is the form taken by the protein into the blood and muscles.

- **Prothrombin and fibrinogen**: When there is a wound, these proteins cause the blood to coagulate and form clots that seal the cut vessels. This is one of the ways your body prevents the complete loss of blood.

- **Carrier proteins**: They are the substances used by the blood for transportation.

Lipids, bodily hormones, medications, etc. do not individually circulate in the blood but are transported by special support with a protein base. For example, the lipoproteins have fat (including cholesterol, which otherwise would stay in the blood vessel wall space), glycoproteins ensure the transportation of sexual hormones in the blood, etc.

- **Pro-inflammatory proteins**: These proteins (cytokines) trigger the defensive reaction of swelling, which allows the tissues to destroy any foreign element that threatens their space.

The liver will not store proteins. It transforms extra protein into urea, which is then sent to the kidneys. This conversion is an effort for the liver.

Continuous protein overloads will eventually stress the liver and cause it to deteriorate.

Metabolism of Fats

The liver synthesizes lipids that are useful to the body, such as phospholipids. It can either send these lipids straight into the blood or store them in its reserves for future needs. Once the liver stores too many fats, which is what happens whenever we eat too much food that contains lipids, it becomes congested with fats, a disorder that can result in fatty degeneration of the liver.

Common factors that can result in a fatty liver include:

- Obesity
- Excess fat in the blood
- Diabetes
- Genetic propensity
- Rapid weight loss
- Side-effect of some medications

Do you know?

Premium treat! The foie gras consumed by gourmets and gastronomes is made out of a liver that has deliberately been congested with body fat when geese are force-fed. This culinary indulgence is made from a diseased liver.

Purification or Cleansing of the Blood

The blood carries numerous toxins, which are the metabolic residues and wastes made by the body while carrying out its duties. The liver is one of the organs responsible for filtering these toxins from the blood to remove them from the body. The liver does this by diluting them in bile, which allows these toxins to leave the body as stool.

Protection against Harmful Agents and Their Destruction

Because of specialized tissues known as Kupffer tissue, the liver destroys everything that threatens the well-being of the body. Elements like germs, toxic elements, carcinogens, carcinogenic cell material, etc. The liver is the only organ in the body that can do this.

How The Liver Works

The liver has an impressive defensive ability as long as it is functioning well. To understand the liver's importance, and how to aid its efforts, it will help to have a detailed explanation of how it works.

Blood Purification

Purification of the blood - the removal of the toxins and poisons it contains is critical because the accumulation of undesirable and injurious materials in the body's cells is the foundation of almost all diseases.

These toxins can wreak havoc when allowed to stay in the body:

- Thicken the blood and clog arteries (cardiovascular diseases)
- Attack the bones (joint disease, rheumatism)

- Clog the respiratory system (bronchitis, colds, asthma, etc.)
- Saturate your skin (acne, eczema, and other pores and skin disorders)
- Form clusters in the organs (such as kidney or bile stones)
- Form debris on the cells (cellulitis, being overweight)
- Alter cells functionality (malignancy)

The filtration and elimination of toxins are done by hepatocyte cells, the basic blocks of the liver. They make up for 80% of the tissues in the liver, while the remaining 20% is the Kupffer cells mentioned earlier concerning their protection against, and damage of any pathogens or other dangerous agents that threaten the body's physical well-being.

Hepatocytes

The liver is crisscrossed by many sinusoidal capillaries that are far away from the portal vein. The total amount of these capillaries is encircled by hepatocytes, which effectively form a coating that envelops every sinusoidal capillary. The wall space of the capillaries is pierced with small "home windows" that allow toxins to leave the blood and meet the hepatocytes. This meeting occurs in the perisinusoidal area between your hepatocytes and the wall space of the capillaries. Referred to as the area of Disse, it is filled with blood.

Microvillae of hepatocytes extends into this space, absorbing the different parts of the sinusoids.

Toxins that come in contact with the hepatocytes have several origins. They can be:

Toxins

- Proteins wastes (urea)
- Wastes from fat (cholesterol, saturated essential fatty acids)
- Poisons caused by intestinal fermentation and putrefaction (indoles, scatoles, etc.)
- Carbohydrate waste material (acids, flocculants, etc.)
- Mineral waste materials (Salt, chlorine, potassium, etc.)
- Hormone waste

- Dead cells (for example, of red blood cells)

Toxic Substances

- Alcohol

- Medications

- Antibiotics

- Heavy metals from pollution color agents and other food additives

- Pesticides

- Tobacco

The purification of the blood by the hepatocytes is an active task. Contrary to the kidneys, where blood vessel filtering happens passively because of the pressure of the blood moving through the renal filtration system, the liver works actively to fully capture toxins and poisons and also to transform their characteristics. Simply put, it actively seeks to neutralize and deactivate them. This makes them harmless to be removed without posing a threat to other parts of the body.

Warning

Alcohol is not food but poison your body looks for ways to expunge by neutralizing it. The liver plays a very important role in cases like this as it neutralizes 95% of the alcohol taken into your body.

Even though you're taking in "a little," you are creating a great deal of work for your liver. For more than a year, daily use of 1¼ glasses of wines with 12 percent alcohol content results in 15 quarts of pure alcoholic drinks.

This transformation and neutralization occur in two stages.

Phase 1

This phase involves transforming harmful substances by using different procedures:

- Oxidation: the material combines mixes o2.

- Reduction: o2 is taken off the substance.

- Hydrolysis: the substance is divided by dilution with drinking water.

These chemical transformations happen due to the work of the enzymes in the hepatocytes. Among the enzymes, one of the most important is cytochrome oxidase P450.

Phase 2

This phase involves the neutralization and deactivation of harmful substances.

The conjugation procedure is used here; this means the toxin or poisonous substance is coupled with another molecule, which has the required characteristics for neutralizing harmful elements. Glucuronic acidity is the most common molecule used to accomplish conjugation. Toxins and poisons which have been neutralized in this manner will then be released by the hepatocytes and other substances to create bile.

The Protection of your body and the Damage of Assailants

Aside from toxins produced by the body's normal functioning-which is a major concern for the hepatocytes-the liver has another special tissue at its disposal to guard itself against both external and internal attacks that threaten the physical health of the body. They are the Kupffer cells mentioned earlier.

Good to know

The cells division of the liver:

- Hepatocytes: 80 percent
- Kupffer cells: 20 percent

Kupffer Cells

Kupffer cells aren't set up like hepatocytes but they are mobile. Their location in the sinusoidal capillaries puts them in direct contact with all the blood that enters the liver because they are effectively immersed in the blood for that reason.

Kupffer tissues are macrophages, they are large in

proportions (macro), and are capable of swallowing and breaking down (phage), they process and eliminate all substances which have not been neutralized and removed by hepatocytes. These injurious elements are mainly:

- Dead or diseased cells
- Cancerous cells (metastatic cells transported by the blood)
- Poorly digested proteins from the intestines
- Bacteria
- Viruses
- Parasites (amoebas, malaria plasmodia, etc.)
- Yeast (Candidiasis)
- Medications
- Unwanted chemical compounds (herbicides, pesticides, antioxidants, preservatives, etc.)
- Synthetic substances
- Carcinogenic substances
- Drugs
- Heavy metals
- Toxins caused by pollution

Good to know

Watch out for foreign protein! While all proteins are made

of the same basic proteins, every living individual has a distinctively unique series of proteins according to each hereditary code. The disease-fighting ability knows how to distinguish between the proteins in the body and the foreign ones, it also destroys any protein it detects as alien: germs, pet secretions (venom), herb tissues (poisons), etc. that are dangerous for the body. Whenever we eat protein (such as those found in seafood or meats), the body identifies it as "other protein" not a personal protein, and therefore breaks it down.

Good to know

"The number of medications now known as hepatotoxic [damaging to liver cells] has grown considerably. This is partly due to the introduction of new substances, but also due to the past recognition of the hepatotoxicity of older medications. "Presently more than six hundred medications are suspected of hepatotoxicity."

Kupffer tissues use enzymes to help them "break down" pathogens. The foreign element is killed if it's a full-time income entity (germ or cells) or destroyed if it's a toxic molecule or substance. In any case, the pathogen is divided into smaller, tiny particles. This way, Kupffer tissue rids the blood of most of these elements.

Kupffer cells have numerous activities to perform, and like all workers, they might need time to break down and recuperate. If they are overworked, which is what happens when different kinds of intoxication are competing (medications, tobacco, drugs, alcoholic beverages, etc.), they are less effective. They only absorb few of the intrusive elements and do not digest them properly. The toxins evade them and make their way deeper into the body.

Kupffer Tissues and the Immune system

There are many types of macrophages in the body, in the bone marrow, brain, spleen, etc. Wherever their location, they contribute to the immune system, whose responsibility is to safeguard the body from the external elements (bacteria, cancerous cells, toxins, etc.). The Kupffer tissues do not work differently from other macrophages situated in the many organs of the body, but they constitute 80 to 90% of the tissue-resident macrophages in the body. Their reputation as powerful defenders is because of their extremely high number. Remember, they represent a substantial portion of the tissue of the liver, an organ already known for its large size! Kupffer cells are the "secret tool" of the liver which makes it a robust defender of the body.

Do you know?

Bacterial infections and yeast constitute a large number of microbes that are harmful to humans, however, the liver can destroy them. The disease-fighting capability is therefore not the only thing to kill microbes; the liver does too.

The significance of the liver is further emphasized as it is the first macrophages blockage encountered by food ingredients, medications, drugs, pollutants, etc. arriving from the intestines. As long as the liver is healthy, these dangerous substances cannot invade your body to gather in the terrain but are destroyed before they can cause any harm. However, when the liver is weak and has been overworked, these substances get into the blood and then yourtissues. Another macrophages of the disease fighting ability then get into action to avoid the degradation of the cells and possible disease. Their ability to defend the body is dependent on the number of toxins that enter the body.

The production of bile for the digestion of fats.

The bile secreted from the hepatocytes is collected by little tubes referred to as the bile canaliculi. These little tubes connect to create larger types that subsequently form the hepatic channel, by which the bile is usually conducted towards the gallbladder and intestines.

The bile plays two different roles:

- It aids the removal of toxins and poisons, which require continuous secretion and constant elimination toward the intestine.
- It aids the digestion and absorption of lipids (fat) in the small intestine, something that requires periodic excretion (in every food).
- There is a need to understand that these two roles of the bile can only be performed with the gallbladder. The bile continually released in the liver can

circulate directly and without interruption toward the intestine bypassing the hepatic and bile ducts, which helps to remove toxins. The gallbladder, in the meantime, in its capacity like a tank can store a particular level of bile, which warranties its periodic release for food digestion.

Bile

The liver releases around one quart of bile daily. This can be a limpid, viscous fluid that contains good alkaline pH (7.six to eight 8.6). Bile is yellowish and has a bitter taste. (This explains why a person who is bitter and upset may be referred to as "a total bile.")

The bile stored in the gallbladder is more concentrated than that which flows straight into the intestine. The color of the bile can be different; it is really olive green.

The different parts of bile are:

- Water
- Bile salts
- Bilirubin
- Cholesterol
- Lecithin
- Various minerals

Bile salts come with an emulsifying action, more importantly, they divide fat into droplets, that allow the pancreatic lipase to break them down completely. This preparation from the bile salts encourages the assimilation of liposoluble (fat-soluble) vitamins - vitamins A, D, E, K, and omega-3 and omega-6.

Whenever there are liver deficiencies, there is poor absorption of fat-soluble vitamins and the symptoms of deficiency illnesses with a decrease in overall health.

Too little bile salts in the gallbladder can lead to weak emulsification from the cholesterol in bile, and therefore a risk of cholesterol solidifying, which can cause gallstones. Bilirubin is a bile pigment or substance caused by the breakdown of blood hemoglobin. It plays no digestive function as it is a waste that needs to be removed. Its brownish-yellow tinge gives stool its color.

In someone who has hepatitis, the bile ducts are congested so much that bilirubin can't flow into the intestines, the stools become colorless, and bilirubin travels into the blood, which gives a yellow tinge to the skin; whites to the eyes and the urine a mahogany color.

Cholesterol is a useful substance but can be harmful when

its level is too high in the body. For this reason, the liver expels cholesterol into the bile when necessary. Because it is not soluble in drinking water, cholesterol cannot be suspended with this liquid. With the ability to maintain a state of suspension system within the bile because of the bile salts and lecithin. If these other substances are missing, the cholesterol particles will precipitate (separate away and clump) and form stones in the gallbladder.

Lecithin is an emulsifier; it helps to create body fat-soluble. Their digestive function is facilitated, which also lessens the chance that they can form debris in the arteries. Lecithin also lowers high blood cholesterol.

Guidelines

Lecithin is gotten from pleasant-tasting granulated pellets and pills. The recommended daily dose of the granulated form is 2 to 4 tablespoons, which may be consumed plain. Granulated lecithin can also be mixed with meals or stirred right into a drink.

The content from the capsules varies from one brand to the other, so it's better to follow the dosage guidelines provided by the manufacturer.

The functions of the Gallbladder

Bile is stored in the gallbladder for digestive system purposes. Once you eat, the food passes through your stomach and goes to the duodenum, where receptors identify the arrival of excess fat. These receptors after that send neural and hormonal signals to the gallbladder asking for the supply of bile that has been set aside for this purpose. The different processes inside play are made up of three steps:

1. Food causes the secretion from the gallbladder. Once the gallbladder is informed of the arrival of fat in the duodenum, it deals 3 or 4 times to evacuate the bile it is has stored. These contractions are usually vigorous, as they are designed to move the bile first with the cystic duct and the bile duct.

2. Postprandial period: The gallbladder will be empty once it has sent its material to the intestines to help digest meals. It remains empty for some time as the bile the liver continues to create is routed not toward the gallbladder but the intestines to also facilitate digestion.

3. Interprandial period: Between foods, the now-empty gallbladder should be refilled to prepare it for the digestion

of another meal. Because the intestine is "fasting" at the moment, it no longer requires any bile to help with the breakdown of food from the previous meal, which includes how well it has worked its way down into the digestive pipe.

Do You Know?

Once the gallbladder has stored much bile and can no longer store and expel bile, surgery must be done to remove the gallbladder. The digestive function will now only be performed by the bile that's continuously released in the liver. Because this implies there is less bile designed for digestion, it's a good idea to eat smaller-sized meals and consume less fat.

The gallbladder refills with bile because of the closing of the sphincter of Oddi, the valve that sets the circulation of bile and pancreatic juice. The bile that is produced by the liver can't enter the intestines, while its forward movement is usually blocked from the sphincter of Oddi. It moves back to the bile and cystic ducts and begins to store in the gallbladder. To reduce the quantity of bile that should be stored, the gallbladder does this by discarding some of its water. Hence, a concentrated and highly active bile is prepared for the arrival of the next meal.

Chapter 2

Liver Detoxification

Liver detox is a process that is meant to cleanse, and get rid of the toxins in your body, to help you lose weight, or enhance your health. You should do all you can to play a dynamic role in your well-being. Your liver is one of the biggest organs in your body. It helps to remove waste materials and deal with various nutrition and medicines.

Most people think a cleanse can extract the toxins from their liver once they drink too many alcoholic beverages or eat processed foods; some think it can revitalize their liver to work better; while many think it can help treat liver disease.

Like most detoxes, liver cleansing has specific steps. You might be required to fast or even to drink only fruit juice or other fluids many times. You may need to consume a limited diet or take natural or health supplements. Some detoxes also necessitate you to purchase a variety of products.

The difference between a Cleanse and Detox?

You may be a bit confused about the difference between the two words "cleanse" and "detoxify", especially since they are used synonymously most of the time.

The primary reason is that most of the techniques in a detoxification plan can also be found in a cleansing plan.

But also for the sake of understanding, let us draw a line between them. The basic difference between them is in the results you would like to obtain.

When you are cleansing your body, you choose to endure a certain process or diet to purge the harmful toxins from your body. Once you choose to endure a cleansing, you eliminate a lot of common foods from your daily diets, such as soft drinks and junks. Whatever contains even a little amount of toxins should be avoided, or else all of your efforts will go to waste.

When you cleanse, you also undergo a certain treatment or diet, but this is for the sole purpose of eliminating waste materials from the body, especially from your digestive tract.

If you choose liver cleansing, you will only need to drink a hot mug of dandelion main tea before going to bed.

Are Liver Detoxes Safe?

There are procedures for liver diseases. But it has not been proven that cleansing diets or supplements can fix liver damage. However, detoxes may harm your liver. Studies have found that accidental liver injuries from organic and health supplements are increasing. Green tea herb, for example, can cause harm like this in form of hepatitis. As well as the coffee enemas used with some regimens can cause bacterial infections and electrolyte issues that might be fatal.

Other things to know about these plans and products:

Some companies use things that can be harmful. Others have made fake claims about how well their products treat serious diseases.

Unpasteurized juices can make you sick, especially if you're old or have a weak immune system.

- When you have kidney disease, a cleanse which involves large amounts of juice can even worsen your illness.
- If you have diabetes, ensure you check with your doctor first before you start a diet plan that will change your eating method.

- If you fast during a detoxification program, you might feel weak or faint, have headaches, or get dehydrated. When you have hepatitis B that has triggered liver harm, fasting can exacerbate the condition.

Does cleansing your Liver help it to heal from Alcoholic beverages or Unhealthy foods?

There isn't any scientific proof that it removes toxins from the body or that it makes you healthier. You might feel better from the detox diet due to the fact you aren't eating ready-made foods with strong fats and processed sugar. These kinds of foods are saturated in calorie consumption but have low nutritional value.

A detoxification diet can also eliminate foods you might be sensitive or delicate to like dairy products, gluten, eggs, or peanuts.

Doctors say liver detoxes aren't very important to your well-being or how well your liver works. There is no evidence that they help to purge toxins from your liver you've taken too many harmful foods or alcoholic drinks.

How to help your liver after taking in too much alcohol

There is a limit on the quantity of alcohol your liver can take in at once. You will be stressing your liver to work harder when you drink too much. And as time goes on, this can lead to inflammation, skin damage, or cancer.

If you must drink alcohol, experts recommend only one drink a day for ladies and two for men. A glass or two is 12 oz. of ale, 5 oz. of wine, or one **ounce** of liquor.

Your liver can heal from small alcoholic damage in days or weeks. More serious harms could take weeks to heal. And if it persists for a long time, it might be long-term damage. Give your liver a break by avoiding alcoholic drinks for at least two days in a row every week.

Does Liver cleansings Protect You From Liver Disease?

Your overall health insurance and your genes affect your liver. So do your daily diet, lifestyle, and environment. Liver detoxification programs don't treat harm or prevent disease.

Ways to prevent liver disease

Lifestyle changes can help to keep your liver healthy

without cleansing programs. These steps are especially important if you are at the risk of liver disease due to heavy alcohol consumption or a family history of liver disease. To prevent liver disease, you should:

- Reduce your alcohol intake.
- Eat well-balanced meals daily. That is five to nine portions of fruits & vegetables, along with dietary fiber from vegetables, nut products, seeds, and whole grains. Ensure to include proteins for the enzymes that help the body detox naturally.
- Keep a healthy weight.
- Exercise daily if you can. Consult with your doctor first if you haven't been exercising in a while.
- Reduce risky conduct that can result in viral hepatitis.
- Avoid leisure drugs. If you must use them, don't share needles or straws to inject or snort them.
- Don't share razors, toothbrushes, or other home items.
- Only get tattoos from a sterile shop.
- Don't have unprotected sex with people you don't know.

Liver cleansing: Truth or fiction?

A healthy liver naturally cleanses itself. A harmed liver can't be helped with liver cleansing. A person with liver disease needs proper treatment and will require lifestyle or diet changes.

Some evidence shows that supplements, such as milk thistle, may improve liver health. However, there is no evidence this supplement will detoxify the liver, or even cure any liver condition.

Liver cleansing also poses some health threats:

- Liver cleansing diets might not offer a balanced diet: A liver cleansing diet might not contain all the nutrition a person requires. And as time goes on, this can lead to deficiencies or malnutrition, especially in children, pregnant women, and people with diabetes and other medical ailments.
- Enemas can be dangerous: Enemas can cause life-threatening harm to the intestines you should administer them correctly.

- Liver cleansing cannot replace treatment: Should a person rely on liver cleansing instead of treatment, serious underlying medical issues can go untreated.

Can cleansing the liver help you lose weight?

Some liver cleansings promise to help with weight reduction by enhancing a person's metabolism. People think that flushing toxins away from the liver can improve metabolism, but there is no evidence to support this claim. Diets low in calories can slow down the body's metabolism. This is because your body adjusts to the reduced nutritional intake by absorbing nutrition more slowly.

Some diets that claim to boost liver health require people to consume few calories for several days. And this may result in short-term weight loss.

A lot of the weight reduction, however, is drinking water weight, which may come back once a person starts to eat normally again.

Chapter 3

How a Detoxification Diet works

In most cases, a person can choose to detoxify when he needs to get over a particular addiction such as drugs, alcohol, smoking, and, even overeating. Detoxification short for "cleansing," is a way of treating poison by neutralizing the toxic properties, and also improving the health of the liver.

Most of the products people use and consume contain certain degrees of "poisons" that are deemed "safe" because the amounts are too insignificant to harm your body.

However, if we constantly use and consume these products we will be building up poisons inside our body without realizing it, and these toxins are difficult, perhaps impossible to eliminate without the help of a detox diet.

A detoxification diet will purify the body's organs and circulatory system and allow it to function effectively. Despite it being unpopular nowadays, it has been used for more than 100 years in different nations around the world.

Note that a detoxification diet is highly restrictive. You will need to avoid a lot of foods and drinks that are known to contain harmful toxins.

Due to its permissive nature, doctors only allow their patients to undergo a cleansing diet plan for a restricted period. Furthermore, it is compulsory for people who have certain medical issues (like diabetes) to consult a doctor before engaging in any kind of dietary plan.

The most common cleansing diet is a 13-day plan. The first three days can be an all-liquid fast which is meant to be drinking water, lemon drink, and tea. After this, you can switch to a 10-day veggie and fruit diet where the portions will be highly managed.

After you've completed the 13-day detox diet program you'll then switch to a Paleolithic diet, which involves strictly eating natural and unprocessed food.

Anyone serious about ridding his/her body of toxins should avoid the following: cigarettes, drugs, caffeine, alcohol, and overly processed food items and supplements. He/she should adhere to eating natural fruits & vegetables, nut products, and grains (whole or natural) because they are guaranteed to get rid of pesticides and other poisons.

Foods like clean drinking water, natural herbs, and lemon juice aid the entire detoxification plan. The largest risk posed by detox diet though is a lack of proteins.

Once you undergo a cleansing diet program, you are also advised to get an entire body cleaning plan. Some people do sauna, or even laxatives or enemas to enhance the effectiveness of these plans.

The Importance of the Liver Cleansing

While detox is broader as it concerns eliminating harmful toxins from the body, a cleanse can be more specific about what part of the body needs to be cleansed. In this guide, the main focus will be on liver cleansing.

Why? This is because it is the liver that acts as the body's first defense against harmful toxins by filtering them out and avoiding their entry into the blood. There are so many things you need to know and understand about how liver cleansing works that it requires to be discussed at length separately. In the next chapter, you will discover how important a liver cleansing is to your health.

Understanding The Liver Cleansing Process

There are many options to choose from when it comes to

cleansing and detox programs. But if you have to choose one specifically, then you might like to consider liver cleansing.

Know Your Liver

The liver weighs approximately 49 oz. (or 1.4 kilograms) and is about 8 to 9 inches (or 20 to 23 centimeters) in size. It is one of the most vital, but basically the most abused organ in the body. Usually, people don't think about it or even value it until it starts to malfunction. Failure to take care of your liver or be conscious of it can lead to serious degenerative ailments that are usually irreversible.

The liver is the body's natural detoxing system. It breaks down toxins and restricts them from entering the blood; produces bile to aid food digestion; stores energy with glucose, and metabolizes fat and proteins.

Once the liver is overwhelmed by overly processed foods that contain high amounts of toxins, preservatives, pesticides, chemicals, and whatnots, it begins to malfunction. Physical symptoms of a damaged liver include high cholesterol and triglyceride levels, malnutrition, gallstones, and allergic reactions.

How Liver Cleansing Works

There are various options for performing a liver cleansing; the basic difference is usually the amount of time devoted to each stage during the process. However, the entire stages are described below.

The first stage of liver cleansing is to fast. This technique is to eliminate any trace of toxins that remains in your system, especially your liver by not eating anything that will refill this "toxic" source. The only things that will go into your system are water and organic teas. This fast will most likely last for 48 hours. In a few variations, many people drink fresh fruit juice such as apple or lemon juice along with specific amounts of essential olive oil and Epsom salts, aside from just drinking water and natural teas.

At the end of the fasting stage, the next phase is to gradually transition back again to solid foods by eating raw vegetables & fruits. You should yourself a break of 7-10 days before re-introducing cooked foods. This will be achieved gradually; you should start with one cooked meal a day. In most variants of the cleanse, this phase demands maintaining the routine of regularly drinking herbal tea, especially dandelion main and dairy thistle.

People who are uncomfortable with carrying out a highly restrictive diet would usually resort to other alternatives for liver cleansing like acupuncture and the use of essential oils, that are either applied on the skin or put into hot tea.

Most people who choose to carry out a liver cleansing will also undergo a colon detox because most experts say that one can't be fully effective without the other. Note that you might feel nauseous or have the urge to vomit or even vomit halfway through your liver cleansing diet due to the drastic change in your daily diet and the purging of toxins from your body.

Also, women who are going to menstruate during the liver cleansing should avoid the diet. This is because the liver does almost double work during this period as it helps to remove excess liquids from your body. Therefore, liver cleansing will only stress the already busy organ.

Advantages of Liver Cleansing

The most obvious benefit you will get from liver cleansing

is a toxin-free liver. It is just like resetting your body back to when you were a healthy young child. A healthy liver also means a stronger disease-fighting ability. You will observe that any previous conditions you might have had before dies, conditions like gall stones, allergies, and hepatitis. The liver cleansing will also regulate your blood sugar and body fat; it will also raise the level of amino acids that get to your cells.

Apart from better overall wellbeing, liver cleansing also can alleviate body pain, nausea, and exhaustion. You will be more energized and happy. Lastly, people who go through the whole liver cleansing process will be able to form healthy habits and overcome certain addictions, which eventually makes them healthier and more disciplined.

Super Foods for the Liver

The section lists food items that will help to improve and maintain the fitness of your liver. It is possible to juice them through the initial stages of your cleansing and eat them uncooked or steamed after you have started introducing food back to your diet. These foods for your liver are broccoli, artichokes, cauliflower, beets, carrots, cabbage, wild greens, and sprouts. These food types contain high levels of fiber, zinc, and nutritional vitamins C and Electronic.

"Anti-Liver" Foods to avoid

Foods that have been processed too much contain many chemicals, additives, and chemical preservatives, hence making them more complicated for the liver to process. Some good examples are sugary foods such as pastries, and foods that contain too much fat and salts, such as French fries, processed foods, and sausages.

You need to limit your intake of caffeine and alcohol, or better still avoid them completely. You should know that alcoholic drinks are one of the primary causes of liver failure.

The Side effects to Expect

Since you now have a good idea of how liver cleansings and detoxification diet works, you can start planning on the diet plan you intend to follow. Remember that it is strongly advised to seek advice from a medical expert before engaging in any kind of extreme procedure, for programs like these can be dangerous.

Before participating in any kind of cleanse or detox, understand that you might experience some side effects. The body has become used to its toxic state that it will at first respond negatively to the cleansing. Certain elements of the body will exhibit strange and often uncomfortable symptoms due to the circulation of toxins that the body is progressively purging. For example, if the toxins are continually being expelled through the skin pores you might develop rashes.

Staining can also happen, even though this is short-term. You can also emit an unusual body odor due to the kind of foods and fluids that you will be consuming for cleansing and detoxification. Long-term cleanse and detox programs will also trigger nausea and fatigue.

Cleansing and detoxification diets that are long-term can also cause substantial weight loss.

Another common side-effect that a lot of people experience during a cleanse and detoxification diet is insomnia. This might happen as a result of the chemical changes and readjustment of hormonal levels that the inner system is experiencing.

The liquid phase in the first stage of the cleansing diet can cause mood swings, so expect to experience some changes in your mood during your cleansing.

Because of these side effects, it is highly advised that you schedule your detox program around when you won't have to stress yourself or undergo any strenuous activity.

Start with the Intestinal tract and Kidney Cleanse

Once you've gathered every item you need, you must first undergo the cleansing diet before you move to the detox diet. Many experts recommend a colon and kidney cleansing before the liver cleansing, if you wish you can consult a doctor about how to do this on your own or conduct some personal research about these other cleanses.

Liver cleansing is the most potent of the three so it's advised your kidneys and intestinal tracts are completely cleared out to reduce the strain in your body.

Variations of the Liver cleansing

To perform the first variance of the liver cleansing, follow the steps below:

Step 1: Prepare lemon fruit juice, either with 3 lemons or even 6 (90 ml) tablespoons of lemon juice.

Step 2: Grate the two 2 garlic cloves and about 2 ins (5 cm) of the new ginger root and blend these thoroughly in the juice concoction. Garlic clove has high detoxifying and anti-bacterial qualities, while ginger increases blood circulation.

Step 3: Put 2 tablespoons (30 ml) of chilly pressed flaxseed essential oil. This contains Omega 3 fatty acids that can stabilize your liver's bile production.

Step 4: Add 1 teaspoon (5 ml) of Acidophilus. It is an important ingredient for liver cleansing; it contains good germs that will stop your liver triglyceride level from rising.

Step 5: Put in a pinch of cayenne pepper to aid your liver in purging the toxins out.

Step 6: Mix everything until it becomes smooth. It should be taken at 2 PM, 6 PM and 8 PM. To avoid blending three times a day, combine 3 times the total amount in the recipe to make 3 servings in a single blend.

Step 7: Through the entire cleansing, eat 1 fruit during breakfast and lunch. Normally, you should not eat anything after 2 PM or once you have started your cleanse.

Anticipate more frequent trips to the toilet during the cleansing because it acts mainly as a laxative.

Do the cleanse over the weekend especially on Sunday to enable you to have time to rest.

To do the other variant of the liver cleansing, follow these steps:

Step 1: Prepare three to four large lemons and squeeze their juice pour 6 to 9 (90 to 105 ml) of lemon juice into a container.

Step 2: Add 4 spoons (60 ml) of Magnesium Sulfate or even Epsom salts into the juice and blend it thoroughly. Epsom salts are a potent laxative that will increase the purging of toxins from your body.

Step 3: Pour into a mug (118 ml) of olive oil. This will assist the gall in the production of bile.

Step 4: Although this is optional, you can pour into the glass a dose of cola, this is to make it easier for you to gulp down the concoction.

Step 5: Mix everything before drinking. Ensure you drink it on an empty stomach. Eat only one fruit at breakfast and lunch. You can eat another fruit by 3 pm, and drink the liver cleansing combination exactly 4 hrs after your dinner, as you have to drink it on an empty stomach

Step 6: You can get 4 Orthinine pills while taking this mixture, although this is another optional step. Orthinine is a non-protein amino acid that will help you to sleep immediately so you don't feel nauseous after drinking the mixture.

This cleansing should be done over the weekend, preferably on Saturday.

Move on to some Liver Detoxification Tea

At the end of the liver cleansing, you need to transition to a healthy lifestyle to be able to maintain the effects of the purge. You need to focus on a liquid diet plan for the next 12 hrs to a day after the cleanse, which comprises strictly clean water and the liver detox green tea.

To prepare the liver detoxification tea, you will need hepatic herbs, which specifically help to improve the general health of the liver. Then dandelion root, prickly ash, dairy thistle, yarrow, fennel, or even yarrow. Other options are the hill grape, hyssop, goldenseal, wild indigo, horseradish, or even motherwort herbs. Note that this mountain grape, dandelion root, and ash herbs also aid the cleansing of your blood and increase your metabolism.

There are lots of tea mixtures that can be used for liver cleansing available in many natural food stores. However, ensure you gather your facts about the manufacturers of the tea beforehand for security reasons.

To prepare the tea, you need to first boil water. The tea won't work if it will be cold or at room temperature. After boiling, steep the herbal tea for 3 to 5 minutes (or according to the manufacturer's instructions, for a few teas have to be steeped for 20 minutes) before you can drink it. You can add a pinch of cayenne pepper or a few drops of freshly squeezed lemon juice.

At the end of the liquid diet plan, gradually move to food. Start by eating one fruit for each meal of the day for the next 24 to 48 hrs. Then introduce more fresh vegetables for the next 24 to 48 hours. After this, move to soft meals like grilled or steamed lean proteins (fish or tofu) before going back again to your normal diet. A lot of people choose to stick to a vegetarian or Paleolithic diet after liver cleansing for health reasons.

A liver cleansing should be done once every year because of its highly potent effects. If you think you need to undergo another cleansing before the end of one year, you should consider a medical doctor for guidance.

Chapter 4

The Idea Of Terrain

The body is a composition of cells, even your organs are clusters of cells. The cell is the essential unit of structure living things. Tissues contain special internal structures called organelles; they have specific duties to produce materials used elsewhere within the cell or in the body. Their activity enables your body to breathe, produce energy, eliminate wastes, reproduce, and receive and send messages.

Do You know?

Cells are built in the same basic model but are different from each other based on their functions. This is one way we can differentiate among the kidney, liver, intestine, bone, muscle, and nerve tissues, red and white blood cells, ova, spermatozoa, etc.

Like every living thing, cells can only survive in a good environment.

In the body this environment is liquid and makes up for 70 % of our body weight, forming what we should call its landscape. The terrain involves various fluids.

A few of these liquids come in direct connection with the tissues:

- Intracells liquid earned its name from its ability to fill the insides of the tissue. Our physical organism is made up primarily of fluid, which represents 50% of the body weight.

- Extra cells liquid, or interstitial liquid, is outside your cells - i.e. in the areas between them. It bathes and surrounds the cell material. Extra cell fluid controls the external environment of the cells and takes about 15% of the body weight.

Other terrain fluids are not in direct connection with the cells:

- Blood circulates in the arteries.

- Lymph moves through the lymphatic vessels.

Combined, these last two fluids take 5% of the body weight.

Do You know?

Only 30% of the bodyweight comprises solid particles, that are primarily nutrient salts: calcium mineral, magnesium, potassium, etc. The highest concentrations of these nutrient salts are found in the skeleton, skull, tresses, and tendons. Nutrient salts play a role in the composition of cell walls, cells, and organs.

Because a cell's success is entirely based on its immediate environment, the composition of the fluids is of critical importance.

Ideal Terrain

There is a perfect composition of the terrain that delivers vitality and maximum strength to the tissues and organs in your body for optimal physical health. A simple consequence of this situation is that any alteration to this composition compromises your health and makes you vulnerable to sickness.

Changes in the structure of the body cells happen primarily because of the components that have been put into their ideal condition. These are elements that are either foreign to the ground but are usually present in smaller amounts (the crystals, urea, etc.) or materials that are not absorbable into the terrain (pollutants, food additives, etc.). This build-up of harmful toxins that overburden the landscape is, by natural medicine, a serious reason behind the disease. The major problem here is excesses, and recovery requires the elimination of these toxins.

The environment can also be disrupted by the lack of substances essential for its ideal growth. These are chemicals such as nutritional vitamins, nutrients, and trace elements that are usually in the environment but for one reason or another, are temporarily insufficient. The main problem here is a deficiency, which may be treated by giving your body the nutrition it lacks, either through diet or supplements.

How Toxins make us sick

When toxins build up in the body, they can make us sick in different ways.

The blood vessels become thicker and are caused by this, it also becomes denser and weightier. And due to this present condition, it can't flow easily through the arteries. Wastes that should normally be transported to the excretory organs by the blood get into the lymph and other cells fluids. The longer this polluted and congested condition lasts, the more toxins that will be released into these fluids.

As time goes on, the cells will swim in a veritable swamp, the inactive mass which paralyzes all exchanges. Materials of o2 and nutrients can't make their way to the tissue, so the cells can no longer perform their duties, neither can the organs they constitute. Wastes accumulate, and this reduces the body's ability to function properly.

The walls of the arteries become filled with wastes, decreasing their size and slowing blood circulation, which affects tissue irrigation and exchange.

The joints become blocked, the kidneys also become blocked and eliminate wastes less effectively, your skin closes up, and the liver becomes congested.

The body's tissues and mucous membranes are irritated by wastes. They become inflamed and in the long run become hardened and sclerotic. They also are more susceptible to infections. Harmful mobile mutations (malignancy) begin to take place.

The harmful implications of toxins are as a consequence of:

- Their mass. They take up so much space that they

hinder and stop the vessels and cells' material.

- Their aggressiveness. They irritate, inflame, and eliminate cells.

Illness Due To An Overload Of Toxins

It is logical to conclude that toxins are the basic element and the starting point of any disease. When confronted with a buildup of toxins, your body does not stay passive but actively tries to get rid of them. Ailments are therefore described as the presence of toxins in the body and the efforts of your body to get rid of these toxins.

For instance, in respiratory sickness, we sneeze, cough, or expectorate to get rid of elements that are constraining the alveoli (asthma), bronchia(bronchitis), tonsils (coughs), sinuses (sinusitis), or nose (common chilly).

All pores and skin disorders are because of the rejection of either acidic substance by the sudoriferous glands (dried out eczema, damaged and chapped skin) or colloidal wastes by the sebaceous glands (acne, comes, greasy epidermis, oozing eczema).

The presence of excess food substances in the intestines

and stomach can cause regurgitation, indigestion, nausea, vomiting, or diarrhea. When these elements are irritating or fermenting, they cause swelling of the mucous membranes of the digestive system (gastritis, enteritis, colitis) or they produce gas

(bloating).

Warning!

Intestinal fermentation and putrefaction produce harmful and annoying substances such as indole, phenol, hydrogen sulfite, methane, and ptomaine, which attack and inflame the mucous membranes of the intestine.

Bones become inflamed, blocked, and painful, and unless treated, they can be severely deformed (arthritis rheumatoid). Regarding gout, sharp, needlelike "crystals" of the crystals deposit may form in a combined or surrounding tissue, causing irritation and injury.

Cardiovascular diseases are caused by the existence of surplus substances (cholesterol, essential fatty acids) that thicken the blood, accumulate in the arteries and thicken the wall space (arteriosclerosis), and inflame the wall space of arteries (phlebitis), which can either deform them (varicose blood vessels) or clog them (heart strike, stroke, embolism).

In renal (kidney) disease, the disturbing substances are protein wastes. In the case of obesity, it is body fat. In diabetes, sugar is a causative agent. Carcinogenic substances are a problem of malignancy, as well as things that trigger allergies in allergic reactions. The poisonous agent in stomach ulcers is gastric acidity.

What is the Foundation of Toxins?

Some toxins in the body are caused by tissue deterioration. The body must continually get rid of the remnants of depleted tissues, the dead red blood vessel cells used nutrient salts, skin tightening and, ammonia, etc. the greater part of toxins resulting from the use of food substances by your body. Proteins produce crystals and urea, blood sugar produces lactic acidity, and fats develop a variety of acids and cholesterol.

The production of the toxins is normal and your body is equipped to eliminate them.

In the case of overeating, the amount of toxins increases far beyond the normal level. Subsequently, in cities where overeating is common, the body consumes and produces an abnormal level of toxins, which eventually exceeds the level of toxins the body is capable of removing.

The toxins which can't be excreted or passed out as waste products stay in the body and begin to build up in the cell surfaces.

What About Toxins?

Toxins shouldn't be in your body. They are foreign elements that harm the body and the organism. All the chemical poisons produced by pollution from the environment, water, and ground (guide, cadmium, mercury, therefore forth) are believed to be toxic substances.

Other harmful foreign materials enter the body through common food chemicals, pesticides, herbicides, and fungicides that are regularly used in industrial agriculture to preserve food crops and pet products. From the four thousand different compounds found in cigarette smoke, such as benzene, uranium, and formaldehyde, the

American Cancer Community says that at least seventy are known to cause cancer, and many others additional health issues. Some drugs and vaccines also contain toxins.

Many of these toxins are difficult to remove because your body is not made to receive or dispose of them. Because of its detoxifying abilities, the liver is the best organ equipped to neutralize and eliminate them.

Classification Of Harmful Toxins And Toxins By Entry Way

Toxins primarily enter the body in three different ways:

Digestive System: Food and Beverage

- Excessive use of sugar, fat, protein, salt, etc.
- Food chemicals: colorings, chemical preservatives, anti-rancidity products, etc.
- Pesticides, herbicides, and fungicides used in agriculture.
- Medications, development promoters, and antibiotics used in the production of animal products.

- Drugs and medications.
- Polluted water and crops

Respiratory Tract

- Polluted air (commercial emissions, automobile emissions, etc.).
- Air that contains excessive particulate matter.
- Tobacco smoke

Skin

- Synthetic and non-organic cosmetic products, talcum and other powders, creams, hair dye, hair shampoo, deodorant, curly hair conditioner, cleaning soap, and other personal care products

Do You know?

Overeating does not only lead to obesity but also exposes you to the vulnerability of harmful substances. However, it is possible to have a buildup of toxins inside your body and still not be overweight.

The Emunctory Organs: Removal of Toxins.

To keep up with the health of the ground of the physiological cell, your body has at its disposal five organs that filter toxins from the blood and expel them from your body. These organs are the liver, intestines, kidneys, pores, and skin (using its sudoriferous and sebaceous glands), and lungs.

These eliminatory organs are technically known as the emunctory organs; they serve as pathways for the removal of toxins from the body.

These organs function normally when they are not overwhelmed with the removal of harmful substances. Besides, they also function as expected when the amount of toxins taken into the body is minimal. The tissues also play their role as expected because the excretory organs are removing the toxins at the same speed at which they're appearing.

Alternatively, when the amount of toxins in the body is too high, the eliminatory ability of these organs begins to reduce and the pathway starts to accumulate higher levels of toxins. Also, if these excretory organs are slow or deficient, the level of toxins in the body will increase, and this will eventually lead to illness.

Draining Toxins

If a disease is triggered by the accumulation of toxins in the body, the most logical thing to do is to get a treatment that will eliminate these harmful substances from the body.

This deliberate removal of toxins is done by draining or purging which is also referred to as detoxification.

Purging involves stimulating the body's various excretory systems to be able to accelerate the speed at which toxins are filtered out of the blood and then carried out your body. This stimulation of the emunctory organs can be done in different ways through the drainers-foods, medicinal natural herbs, massage, hydrotherapy that are used to intensify the eliminatory abilities of the emunctory organs.

The emunctory organs are essential in draining toxins from the body and in ridding the body of harmful substances. In treatments that concentrate on intensifying the purging of your body, all efforts are concentrated on these organs.

When the body cannot eliminate all these substances, the next thing to be done is for the body to build a standard for the removal of these toxic materials or to temporarily accelerate the emunctory organs to make up for the delay. One important feature of the draining treatment is the reduction of wastes by the emunctory organs. <u>This increase in elimination should be readily apparent</u>:

- Wastes removed by the intestines could be more abundant or removal will occur more frequently.
- Urine becomes darker because it is discharged alongside wastes and it increases in quantity.
- Your skin will perspire more profusely.
- The respiratory system will release colloidal wastes that have been congesting it.

There will be a consistent reduction in the level of toxins in the tissue. Gradually, the mobile terrain will be clean again, hence, the symptoms of the disease will reduce and then disappear gradually. The organs in the body at this point will be able to carry out their duties effectively because they are no longer congested with toxins.

These organs are quick to recover based on the level of damage the toxic substances have caused and then also on their ability to regenerate.

The role of the Liver

The liver is one of the five excretory organs in the body. The liver is not more important than the other four organs; basically, the five organs are required to be in good condition and work actively together to guarantee good health. However, the functions of the liver differ from that of these other organs.

Similar to the other emunctory organs, the liver removes a large number of toxins. Asides from the removal it also neutralizes harmful toxins. The other four excretory organs don't have this ability, or should we say to the degree to which the liver performs this function (if they will neutralize toxins, they have a lower ability to do it compared to the liver).

Warning

Although the liver has the responsibility of ridding the body of poisons and toxins, it can still be overwhelmed by these substances. Hence, if any excretory organ must maintain its active service and be in good working condition, it must be the liver. Also, whenever it is required for a person to activate an excretory organ due to bad body function, often, the most appropriate organ is the liver.

The liver absorbs a lot of toxic materials in the process of filtering the foreign elements that enter the body. If these elements when absorbed by the liver begins to affect its efficiency, then steps to detoxify the liver must be taken immediately to avoid affecting the performance of other organs in the body.

Summary

- The disease is caused by a build-up of toxins.
- The liver is one of the major organs for eliminating these harmful substances.
- The liver can neutralize both toxins and poisons.

Chapter 5

Liver-Loving Herbs

The liver loves anything bitter. People around the world have long used natural bitter herbs to cleanse the liver, especially after a cold winter. Wild herbs, such as artichoke, dandelion greens, endive, garlic clove, lettuce, radicchio, and onion, were commonly harvested and dried for later use.

All bitter herbs help the functionality of the liver and enhance the secretion of bile.

Unfortunately, most of these green herbs lose their bitter characteristics through hybridizing. The common lettuce, for example, is good without nutrients, but they have a long shelf life. Due to modern food marketing and submission tactics, Western cultures now tend to like lettuce and dislike bitters. But our anatomies need bitters, and herbs are the best places to get them.

Medicinal Herbs

Natural herbs that are ideal for cleansing the liver include celandine, goldenseal, dairy thistle, rue, and wormwood.

Natural herbs are synergistic; this means they rely on each other to work. Medicinal natural herbs are best used incompatible mixtures and limited to intervals. Choose a plan and stick to it for three to six weeks, or change your daily combinations to suit your needs.

Herbs can be used in capsule form or as green tea potions that can be taken during the day. The traditional recipe for Swedish bitters is a mixture of eleven herbal remedies that have been used effectively for hundreds of years. It is sold in natural food shops as a packed blend, but you can also buy the dried herbs, mix them yourself, and brew your Swedish bitters tea as you like.

You can prepare a potion by pouring hot water on the dried herbs and allowing it to steep for 5 minutes or more before sieving out the liquid and then drinking. Berries can be steeped the same way, but roots and barks should be boiled for five to fifteen minutes to activate their active nutrients. If you are using a mixture of bark, berries, and root base, you should first pulverize them into powder with a spice mill or coffee grinder, then take the powdered mixture or teaspoon or pour hot water over it and allow it to steep before drinking.

Make liver-friendly herbs a normal part of your liver cleansing routine. It is especially important to have a mixture of liver herbs once you feel weak, eaten too much, had a drinking spree, feel stressed out, or fatigued. Anise, fennel seed, ginger, licorice main, and peppermint make mixtures (teas) that have enjoyable flavor and aids the breakdown of the substances.

 Use one of these as a taste enhancer along with three or four bitter herbs. These herbs are mostly available in natural food stores and can be turned into green tea. Don't add any sweetener; just drink the tea just like the medication it is. Herbal treatments that help the liver are usually bitter; that is why they are effective for cleansing. Taking them with an aromatic herb can reduce the potency of the medicine.

Therapeutic plant juices are also sold by natural food stores. Those that specifically support the liver include dark radish juice, dandelion fruit juice, and nettle fruit juice. Artichoke is a relative of the thistle family and a natural liver tonic; it stimulates the production and circulation of bile and aids the detoxification process.

Culinary Herbs

The use of herbs in cooking continues to become trendy given that chefs understand the wonderful features of the common plants. Culinary herbs are not only the oldest but they are also reputed as one of the most popular taste enhancers, given that they originate from nature and not from the laboratory. Fresh herbs are always the best to use, and they are now always available, even all through winter. There is a nutritional advantage in using fresh herbs over the dried ones that have sat on spice racks for a long time.

The East Indian families, the custom is to place herb seeds, such as anise, dill, and caraway, on the table to chew during or after meals as an aid for the digestive system. Peppermint is also used to ease both the stomach and digestive tract. Use natural lots of natural herbs creatively when preparing your meals.

Fresh herbs can be kept for a couple of weeks in the freezer when covered in a damp paper towel and then placed in a plastic or a container. Aside from tasting delicious, herbal treatments contribute to your overall wellbeing and promote a healthy liver.

Below are a few combinations of vegetable-and-herbs that will support your liver and help you cook your meals to perfection:

- **Beets**: basil, bay leaf, cardamom, dill, marjoram, oregano, tarragon
- **Brussels sprouts**: basil, caraway, dill, savory, thyme
- **Cabbage**: caraway, celery seed, dill, summertime savory, tarragon
- **Carrots**: basil, dill, marjoram, parsley, thyme
- **Cauliflower**: dill, rosemary, summer season savory, tarragon
- **Cucumber**: basil, savory, tarragon
- **Green Coffee Beans**: basil, dill, oregano, rosemary, thyme
- **Onions**: basil, oregano, thyme
- **Peas**: basil, dill, mint, oregano

- **Potatoes**: basil, chives, dill, marjoram, mint, parsley

- **Spinach**: oregano, rosemary, tarragon • squash: basil, dill, oregano, savory

- **Tomato Vegetables**: basil, bay leaf, oregano, parsley

Planning the Liver-Cleansing Menu

For many people, planning healthy meals can be a disruption of their ingrained habits. Write down your exact diet goals. It'll be easier to stick to them when you read them every day.

Fresh Vegetable Juice

A healthy liver is are caused by a normal food diet that is balanced with nutrients.

Vegetables help to cleanse and build the liver. You should use fresh veggie juice, they are easy to break down and quickly deliver a healthy dose of minerals and vitamins to your body. Drink at least eight ounces of fresh fruit juice daily. You should "chew up" the vegetable juice to be able to stimulate your salivary glands and start the digestive system process. The more you include veggie fruit juice in your diet, the easier it will be for your liver to function normally.

Beets, cabbage, carrots, celery, cucumbers, and spinach are easy to juice and can be used in various mixtures. My favorite blend is apple company, carrot, and celery fruit juice with just a little ginger for extra taste and this is because of its liver-loving properties. But since I now consider freshly pressed juice medicine as food, I include some bitter greens: dandelion leaves, endive, and radicchio. Radish, especially dark radish, using its sharp, bitter advantage, is also a great liver stimulant. I also made it a point of duty to regularly add beets to my juice. They are perfect blood cleansers.

I mentioned a compatible mixture in the recipe section to help you get started if juicing is not your thing, nevertheless, you can make your own combinations which will be based on your preference, what is available, and what will facilitate the cleaning process. Cabbage, lettuce, radish, and spinach are juice-able. Wild greens, such as dandelion, lamb's quarters, and pigweed, are available to most people; use them if you are sure they haven't been sprayed with pesticides.

Juicing 3 times a day is recommended if you have the time. You can chill your juice to preserve its freshness for up to two days. Put containers of fresh fruit juice in the fridge until the fruit juice is approximately 40°F, but ensure you don't allow it to freeze. Using an infrared thermometer makes it easier to check up on it. You can fix your juicing routine into your daily life, but it's better to adjust your lifestyle to suit what's best for your liver.

Breakfast

The body has properly fasted after dinner which you had at six o'clock the previous day. Your liver has been allowed to perform its duty of detoxification at night, and you also wake reinvigorated as you practically bounce out of bed! The nourishment the liver requires at this time of the day is half a glass of lemon juice, and 2-3 other glasses of drinking water, and perhaps a mug of liver-cleansing tea-without sweetener. Then take a walk for an hour, or spend half an hour working-out and the remaining 30 minutes jogging. In summer, weed your garden; during winter, spend one hour in the community pool or at the gym. It's enjoyable walking in the fresh air throughout the year, regardless of the weather.

After the exercise, you can have your first meal, ensure it is light. You can take your fresh veggie juice now or eat some fresh grapefruit or other fruits. If you want something bigger, this is the best time to munch down a plate of muesli or cooked dark brown rice cereal, buckwheat cereal, millet cereal, or oatmeal.

Muesli

Muesli is an uncooked food usually served as breakfast, it is made out of grains and fruits, specifically soaked oat flakes and grated apple. It is popular among many Europeans for years and is currently a staple food in North America. If you make your muesli instead of buying it packed from the supermarket, you can have control over the ingredients and include your favorites while avoiding any added sugar.

You don't have to eat only muesli for breakfast, however, it is a healthy snack that can be taken any time of the day; you can even include it in your lunchbox for a midday treat. Follow my recommendations for making homemade muesli with the recipe for Bircher Muesli with Sesame

Seeds, or you can make your version with oats, chopped nut products, berries, peaches, and grated apple company. Add lemon fruit juice and nut dairy to moisten.

Midday Meal

If you are at home, you're in a position to prepare this most significant meal.

If you're at work, you'll probably have to prepare your lunch ahead and take it with you. Take fresh fruits for a salad, along with cooked grains and some toppings or condiments. The noon meal should be unhurried and relaxed. Avoid eating an instant light lunch as it implies that you hurried your meal at the dining table, and might be hungry soon enough.

Main Dishes

For most people, dinner is the most important meal of the day, as it is a time when everyone will be home and can make and talk about food together. Ensure you complement your primary meal with a salad of raw greens or grated vegetables. Understand that at least 75% of your daily diet should contain natural (uncooked) foods.

A Healthy Liver for life

Stick to the liver-cleansing diet for at least twenty-one days or more, but preferably for three months.

Afterward, you might feel so fit that you'll want to stick to the diet plan and neglect your previous diet plan. Once your liver has released its harmful substance, the improvements in your health will be obvious, you will no longer feel weak. Your liver can handle a periodic indulgence, but only as long as liver detoxification becomes a lifestyle.

Chapter 6

The Effects of Alcohol on the Liver?

Alcohol can trigger long-term damage and harm to the liver, especially in people that drink excessively or those that have been drinking for a very long time.

Alcoholic drinks damage the liver by first storing excess fats in the liver. This stage is called alcoholic fatty liver disease. This condition can lead to alcoholic hepatitis, or irritation and inflammation of the liver. Inflammation of the liver leads to irreversible scarring of the organ or cirrhosis.

While the accumulation of extra fat and swelling are usually reversible, the skin damage it eventually causes isn't.

A scarred liver has irreparable liver harm with long-term effects which can be fatal.

What is Alcoholic Fatty Liver Disease (AFLD)?

Alcoholic fatty liver disease (**AFLD**) might be the first stage of liver disease. In AFLD, fats get deposited into the liver tissues, thus harming them. A lot of people who drink heavily over a long period are prone to AFLD. There are two forms of fatty liver disease:

- Non-alcoholic fatty liver disease, or NAFLD: Of the two conditions, NAFLD is not considered to be linked with the consumption of alcohol. However, doctors are currently uncertain about the cause of NAFLD. Although occasionally the disease is moderate, it can, however, worsen in some individuals. Studies are yet to prove whether it is safe for someone with NAFLD to take alcohol in low quantities. Consequently, you must consult with your doctor about your condition to find out if a moderate intake of alcohol is safe for you or not. You should however desist from heavy drinking with NAFLD.

- Alcoholic fatty liver disease, or alcoholic steatosis:

When you have alcoholic fatty liver disease, the cells in your liver start to build-up with an excessive amount of unwanted fat. Drinking alcohol causes your body to create excess fat, and also prevents it from eliminating some of the extra fat you might have. All this extra fat will then be deposited in your liver cells, where it can cause damage. Some fats can even move from other parts of your body to your liver are caused by drinking.

Signs & Outward indications of AFLD

Unfortunately, AFLD only has a few signs and symptoms. The basic symptoms of AFLD are:

- Tiredness
- Experiencing discomfort in your upper abdomen
- The skin begins to take on a yellow color or the excessive whiteness of the eyes.
- Because AFLD has only a few symptoms, it might be difficult for doctors to diagnose in its early stages. AFLD is often diagnosed when a scan is being conducted, or when you undergo a blood test. And this is what reveals the issues with the chemical

substances in your liver.

- Sometimes, doctors cannot discover alcoholic fatty liver disease until it advances into a more threatening condition like cirrhosis.

Treatment of AFLD

ALFD is mainly treated based on the changes that take place in your lifestyle. These changes range from:

- Quitting alcohol completely
- Eating a healthy diet plan
- Weight loss, if you're overweight
- Exercise, which might reduce the amount of fat in the liver

Getting vaccinations such as hepatitis A, hepatitis B, pneumonia, and yearly influenza (flu) shot will not treat AFLD but can help to prevent more serious disorders from happening later on. Also, it is important to consult with your doctor before getting any vitamins, natural herbs, or dietary supplements because some of these diets can further worsen your liver condition.

What is Alcohol Hepatitis?

Alcoholic hepatitis is an inflammation of the liver, and the regular consumption of alcohol can aggravate the situation. The swelling disrupts the liver's regular functions and may lead to several distressing and possibly deadly symptoms.

Symptoms & Factors behind Alcoholic Hepatitis

Some cases of severe alcoholic hepatitis might not have any symptoms, and people who have this disease might not know until it becomes complicated. Some of the likely symptoms include:

- Confusion due to the buildup of toxin ammonia.
- The stomach begins to swell – this is caused by the liver's inability to produce enough of the protein known as albumin.
- Bleeding – this may be serious when the liver cannot produce enough proteins required for blood clotting.
- Bleeding in the throat due to weak arteries that are usually common with hepatitis
- The skin takes on a yellow color and the eyes also become whitish – this is known as jaundice. It happens once the liver cannot breakdown a material

called bilirubin. The jaundice alcoholic hepatitis leads to is not particularly harmful, however, it can imply that there are other harmful underlying liver conditions.

People who have jaundice should get immediate health care.

Scientists are not particularly sure about how alcohol triggers alcoholic hepatitis, but it is known that heavy alcohol plays a significant role. Without taking alcohol, there is no risk of being prone to alcoholic hepatitis. When a person ceases to consume alcohol, the irritation caused by alcoholic hepatitis may eventually go away completely.

Other risk factors that can increase the chances of being prone to alcoholic hepatitis when **coupled** with alcohol misuse include:

- Poor nutrition.
- Disease fighting ability.
- Viral illnesses, especially hepatitis B or hepatitis C.
- Use of Tylenol, especially for an extended period.
- Being older than 55.

- Female gender.
- Obesity.

Dealing with Alcoholic Hepatitis

Treating alcoholic hepatitis requires stopping alcohol intake as this helps the liver to heal faster. Quitting alcohol is the first step to seek in healing your liver, and as more alcoholic drinks are consumed, the liver starts to swell. The good news is that as time goes on, the inflamed liver can even start to reduce as soon as you stop pressuring it with alcoholic drinks.

There are drugs available to stop or reduce irritation. The most common drug used to treat alcoholic hepatitis is steroids. These drugs reduce swelling and suppress the body's disease-fighting ability. They can also be used to reduce recuperation time.

While malnutrition might play a minor role, having a healthy and nutritious diet plan while maintaining a healthy weight has been proven to suppress the symptoms of alcoholic hepatitis.

Unfortunately, the irritation can lead to scarring, which is also known as alcoholic cirrhosis. This skin damage can't be reversed and can have more long-term effects.

What's Cirrhosis?

When you drink excessively, especially for a long period, the healthy cells in your liver are replaced with scar tissue formation. Cirrhosis is the scarring of the liver. Cells in the affected area usually cease to work effectively or even stop working completely.

The more you drink, the higher the chances of damaging your tissue scars and the faster cirrhosis progresses.

And what ultimately happens is that your liver stops working effectively as the efficiency in its operation drops. However, it is not everyone who drinks excessively or that abuses alcohol comes down with cirrhosis. And for people who have cirrhosis, this condition can have severe effects and lifelong consequences.

Causes & symptoms of Alcoholic Cirrhosis

Cirrhosis can have various symptoms that may range from irritation to potentially deadly. Probably the most serious of the symptoms are usually coloration of the eyes and skin, excessive bleeding, and swelling.

The coloration of the eye and skin: The skin begins to take on a yellow color while the eyes also begin to change their color to something whitish (this condition is known as jaundice). It is a serious sign of alcoholic cirrhosis. Jaundice implies a malfunctioning liver, that inevitably leads to an accumulation of toxins that can are deadly. Anyone who has jaundice should get immediate medical care.

- Increased bruising or bleeding: Increased bleeding happens are caused by the liver's inability to produce sufficient components required for blood clotting. Also, it can cause a person to bleed more than they ought to. This symptom is dangerous. After all, a simple bleeding can lead to the loss of huge amount of blood because the bleeding can't be stopped easily. If you notice that you might have increased bleeding, you need to get medical care as soon as possible.

Swelling in the belly, feet, legs, or even ankles: The last important symptom of alcoholic cirrhosis is swelling, especially in the abdomen. This swelling, also known as ascites, happens once the liver can no longer produce the protein that keeps absorbing fluid in the veins. This means that the liver is not working as it should. Accumulation of fluid in the tummy can result in serious health issues.

- Other symptoms include weakness, and exhaustion, decreased appetite, weight reduction, muscle atrophy, nausea or vomiting, discomfort and tenderness in the upper abdomen, an increase in the number of tiny visible arteries on your skin, itchy pores and skin, hair loss, or fever.

Alcoholic cirrhosis is a progression of liver harm, typically beginning as fatty liver disease, which leads to inflammation and then liver scarring. About 35% of heavy drinkers have alcoholic hepatitis, significantly increasing the chance of alcoholic cirrhosis.

Dealing with Alcoholic Cirrhosis

The scarring caused by cirrhosis is usually irreversible,

and will steadily worsen as more alcohol is consumed.

Avoiding alcohol is crucial to stop the development of alcoholic cirrhosis.

Treating any underlying medical condition that can trigger the disease is also important. Illnesses such as hepatitis or a weak immune system may worsen with alcoholic cirrhosis. Maintaining a high-protein, high-calorie diet plan will mostly be recommended by doctors, and also with having a healthy workout system. This activity will optimize the rest of the function of the liver.

Dealing with the complications that arise from cirrhosis is also an essential part of the treatment. Since cirrhosis can't be reversed, its effects must be handled as they unfold.

Usually, the only way to completely get over alcoholic cirrhosis is by having a liver transplant. While a transplant can lead to full recuperation, this option is often not readily available to many people.

To be eligible for a liver transplant for alcoholic cirrhosis, patients must show a certain amount of sobriety so as to ensure that the new liver will not go through the same strains that initially triggered the cirrhosis.

How do you repair Liver damaged by alcohol?

There are several steps you can take to reverse the consequences of alcohol on your liver, such as:

1. **Stop drinking**: If you have been diagnosed with liver disease, the first and most important thing to do is to stop drinking alcohol.

2. **Make other healthy commitments**: This implies that you should stop smoking cigarettes and start to maintain a healthy weight. Similar to alcohol, obesity is one of the leading causes of liver disease, while cigarettes also contain toxins that worsen liver damage.

3. **Watch what you eat**: You should desist from eating many processed foods, sugar, and foods saturated in fats. This helps the liver to avoid unnecessary stress by metabolizing these foods first. A healthy diet plan can as well lead to a healthy liver.

4. **Exercise regularly**: Aside from helping to prevent obesity, exercising can help the liver in different ways. Regular exercise enhances the disease-fighting ability of the liver and reduces the chance of liver malignancy.

5. **Be careful of the kinds of drugs you take**: Some over-the-counter drugs can be harmful to your liver when used in excess, such as acetaminophen.

6. **Don't allow unnecessary toxins into your body**: Avoid illegal drugs; those that are used without prescription and chemicals that contain some amount of toxicity can help to maintain the health of your liver. This implies that you must take the necessary precautions, such as using a face mask when using aerosol sprays, aerosol paints, squirt insecticides, aerosol fungicides, and any type of sprayed chemical substance. You should know those chemicals that are dangerous to your skin and vice versa. And you should use hand gloves when necessary.

Liver Illness & Pancreatitis

Similar to knowing the effect of alcohol on the liver, it's also vital to consider how alcoholism leads to pancreatitis. There is severe pancreatitis and chronic pancreatitis.

The pancreas is a gland behind the stomach in charge of releasing digestive system enzymes and works with the liver to process substances. A swollen pancreas is called pancreatitis.

Acute pancreatitis is a sudden onset swelling that is temporary. The outcomes of the problem range considerably, from being mild, to unpleasant and then deadly, but it's a condition most people recover from. Chronic pancreatitis has more severe symptoms like regular pain, weight reduction, and a possibility of being prone to diabetes.

In nearly all cases, alcohol leads to acute pancreatitis, although other notable causes can include trauma, metabolic conditions, or infections. Often, prolonged alcoholism makes up about 60-90% of chronic pancreatitis cases.

Having chronic pancreatitis puts you at an increased risk of other serious illnesses, like cancer and diabetes. Quitting alcohol increases your chances of dealing with pancreatitis.

Chapter 7

Diseases of the Liver

The liver, like any organ, can be diseased. The illnesses that afflict it are primarily because of loads of work imposed on it through overeating, chemical pollution of meals, alcoholic beverages, drug abuse, and stimulants.

Liver Deficiency

In the case of hepatic deficiency, the liver is not only damaged, but it is also not working as it should. It is poor and lethargic, and hence it is referred to as "sluggish liver." Once the liver is in this state, it is congested, meaning that blood vessels and toxins are stagnating in it. This congestion slows the production and secretion of bile. A sluggish liver can be pretty much pronounced, with regards to the individual. These can cause a lot of medical problems and may affect every part of your body, as almost any hepatic deficiency will inevitably result in an overload of toxins inside the terrain, which is the starting place for disease. However, the first symptom to be noticed is in the digestive system sphere. They are probably the most visible and easiest to detect.

A person who has hepatic deficiency won't be necessarily affected by most of these issues, but usually, a number of them are relevant:

- Difficulty digesting fat (eggs, lotion, high-fat meals, etc.)
- Digestive troubles generally
- Rounds of nausea
- Swelling and sensation heavy round the belly
- Gas or bloating
- Sticky tongue
- Bad breath
- Lack of appetite
- Fatigue and inadequate enthusiasm
- Yellow tinge to your skin and eyes
- Constipation
- Gallstones
- Itching on your skin
- Hemorrhoids

Small hepatic deficiency isn't severe but will impair the quality of life. Someone with this problem may constantly deal with digestive disorders and become weak often and also deal with vitality and enthusiasm. It is only when the deficiency is severe that the cell wall starts to breakdown and other organs become affected.

Bile Stones

The liver is constantly producing bile. While one part of this bile will be carried straight into the intestines from the bile duct, the rest - a little significantly less than half-is set aside inside reserve within the gall bladder to be used for the digestive function of another meal. To reduce the quantity of bile being stored, the mucous membranes from the gallbladder reabsorb a portion of the water it contains, taking the bile's level of water content from 97.5 percent down to 87 percent. At this time, the concentration of solid substances in the bile obviously increases. For example, the quantity of bile salts goes from 1 percent to 6 percent. The composition of bile in the liver is, therefore, not the same as that of the bile stored in the gallbladder, which is 4 to 5 times more concentrated, stringy, and viscous. The big viscosity of gallbladder bile is beneficial for digestion since it has higher articles of digestive fruit juices. However, it can expose the given individual to one danger: the saturation stage is close, and at that point, the ingredients suspended inside will precipitate and form bile stones.

Overeating majorly causes the formation of bile stones.

Meals that are too high and too frequent can degrade the gallbladder. Its walls will also lose their firmness. The bile this organ contains will be ejected imperfectly into the intestine during meals. Some of the bile will remain in the gallbladder, hence, it is prone to have its level of concentration increased. This way, over time, the gallbladder will retain a share of stagnant bile. The cholesterol and nutrient salts it contains will eventually precipitate. This is what happens when a substance that is a liquid solution becomes strong and solidifies. The salts and cholesterol that have been dissolved and suspended in the bile will drop below the organ.

At first, these substances are isolated, but ultimately they are linked with emotions.

This state is normally referred to as biliary sludge i.e. thick bile that can lead to the formation of tiny crystals and then bile stones that may grow to several centimeters in proportions.

Bile stones are not naturally harmful, but by storing within the gallbladder they hinder its proper functioning.

Once the bile necessary for digestion is no longer getting into the small intestine in regular quantities, there is a problem with the digestive system. The solid bile that is stagnating in the gallbladder irritates the mucous membranes, which leads to inflammation and sclerosis. The environment this creates is particularly vulnerable to infection. The worst danger, however, will be when a bile stone leaves the gallbladder. If it's bigger than any part of the bile duct or cystic duct (which connects the gallbladder and the bile duct), it can be stuck in one of these two tubes. This can cause serious pain (liver colic) and contamination of a part of the liver (hepatitis or even jaundice).

Good to know

The formation of bile stones starts with the presence of sludge or thick bile that precipitates and forms crystals. When these microparticles clump together, they form bile stones.

Types Of Hepatitis

Hepatitis attacks are usually liver inflammations. They are considered as severe disorders, seen due to their intensity and generally brief duration. Throughout a hepatitis attack, the liver tissue is inflamed. They crush the bile ducts, which block the circulation of bile and prevents it from passing into the intestines. A few of this clogged bile stagnates in the liver, hindering its detoxifying functions. The others get into the blood. Because it contains many toxins, once it begins to circulate through the blood it can ultimately poison your body.

Hepatitis symptoms have become easy to understand. They are primarily linked to bilirubin, the yellow pigment in bile, which throughout this illness is dispersed through the entire body. They consist of:

- Yellowish coloration, or jaundice (from the French word for yellow: Jaune) of the skin as well as the whites from the eyes
- Darker urine (the normal yellow color of urine is due to the current presence of bilirubin)
- Discolored stools (because they are not getting required the bilirubin they usually get through the

bile carried to the intestines)

Somebody with hepatitis also suffers:

- Fatigue
- Lack of appetite
- Episodic fevers
- Itching

Hepatitis might lead to many things, including something that irritates the bile ducts and causes swelling that obstructs and clogs them. Its various forms are usually the following:

- **Viral hepatitis**: The attack is caused by a virus.
- **Harmful hepatitis**: The attack is caused by poison or medication.
- **Mechanized hepatitis**: A bile stone blocks the bile ducts.
- **Hemolytic hepatitis**: There is an excessive amount of hemoglobin to be broken down (often due to incompatibility of blood types among mother and child, or are caused by blood transfusion).

Did You know?

The liver can be affected by various kinds of viral hepatitis. There are three predominant types, all of which are identified by a different letter.

- Hepatitis A: This is transmitted via water or food that is washed with contaminated water (for example salad greens, raw vegetables, fruits, or shellfish). Hepatitis A is normally for a short period and heals without complications.

- Hepatitis B is transmitted through the blood and can be passed on through the use of unsterilized syringes and other contaminated devices (fine needles). Also, it can be transmitted through sexual interactions. And can be cured without major complications.

- Hepatitis C can be transmitted through the blood. Hepatitis C is problematic as it can turn into a debilitating chronic issue.

Cirrhosis

After the liver has suffered repeated and continuous assaults over a period, lesional disorders happen. Cirrhosis in any form is a severe and chronic disease, caused are caused by a part of the liver being attacked. The damage of cells causes first lesions, after that scarring (fibrosis). Usually, the liver's ability to regenerate is high, however, in the chronic stage, this regeneration cannot happen properly. It generates an excessive amount of fibrous tissue that hardens the liver and slows down cell exchange. The effect is undoubtedly a disruption of the liver's function. The organ will not be able to carry out its duty of protection, cleansing, and bile production, along with many other functions.

Warning

Cirrhosis is the result of a lifestyle that has no respect for that liver. 70% of most cirrhosis diseases are usually due to alcoholism.

The appearance of the liver changes completely. Rather than being smooth, firm, along with heavy brown color, its surface becomes pitted. It becomes rough and takes on a red color. The word cirrhosis originates from this color; in Greek, kirros means "reddish."

Several Diseases Due To Poor Liver Functioning

When the liver stops functioning properly, it not only affects the liver but also other organs that are not even close to the liver.

The Digestive System

The first problem encountered with a damaged liver happens in the digestive system, which makes it obvious that there is a direct link between the liver and this system.

Indigestion

Around the digestive (rather than removal) level, the role played by the liver is in two ways. To begin with, bile emulsifies body fat, breaking them into tiny particles that may end up being attacked by the digestive system juices from the pancreas and intestines. If this first stage is not properly done, fats that are not adequately transformed can cause bouts of nausea or vomiting, a feeling of heaviness, and a sensation that your food did not digest.

The other way the liver plays a vital role in digestion is by alkalizing the alimentary bolus, the size of food from the last meal that is passing through the gastrointestinal tract. To be able to digest protein, the stomach secretes acidic digestive juices. Once the first alimentary bolus exits the stomach it contains a pH of 2.5. Nevertheless, the pancreatic and intestinal fruit juices that are mixed up in intestines can be effective within the alkaline environment i.e. using a pH above 7. The liver is in charge of altering the pH from the alimentary bolus to the particular level needed by these digestive system juices to operate efficiently. The bile produces a high alkaline, having a pH that runs from 7.6 to 8.6. This alkalizes the alimentary bolus and in this manner encourages the complete and efficient digestion of fat. However, if a person is suffering from liver insufficiency, this alkalizing exercise will never be sufficient. The excess fat will stay poorly digested and many digestion disorders will arise.

Constipation

Constipation is commonly believed to be caused by inadequate roughage, lack of exercise, and lack of adequate water. But a generally overlooked cause of this condition is a liver deficiency.

A slow liver can't release adequate bile, and some of the qualities of bile are needed to stimulate intestinal peristalsis, which aids the digestion of food in the digestive tract. So it's not the only soluble fiber that causes contraction in the intestinal muscle tissue but also bile. An adequate secretion of bile allows the stools to move with the intestines even though there is a little bit of insufficient roughage in the dietary plan.

When the bile is too small, the activities of the intestines are slowed down. The partially digested matter remains stagnant and starts to accumulate, which makes the duty of the peristaltic muscle groups more difficult. That is when constipation becomes an issue.

Bile also plays the role of lubricant, making the feces moist and slippery, which hugely facilitates progress with the intestines. It stops the stool from sticking to the mucous membranes in the intestinal wall space, which may also be made slippery by bile. Which means that the feces can move out easily.

Too little bile, alternatively, helps make stool sticky,

which hampers its progress.

Blood and the Circulatory System

After the digestive tract, the blood vessels and circulatory system are most likely to be adversely affected by the hepatic deficiency. Wastes that have been poorly neutralized rather than eliminated by the liver gather in the blood

and form deposits around the vessel walls. On the list of illnesses this can cause, we found the following.

High Cholesterol

All the extra fat we eat goes into the liver. Your body uses just a portion of this quantity, and the rest is transformed into cholesterol, and triglycerides the liver will expel into bile. The product after that goes into the intestines, from where it is normally ejected from the body as a stool when there is sufficient roughage (wholegrain husks, plant materials of fruits & vegetables) to fully capture it.

Fiber is vital for transporting cholesterol around the body. It acts like a fine-mesh internet that traps it. When there is inadequate dietary fiber, the cholesterol will never be trapped and will be reabsorbed by your body. If you don't have sufficient fiber in

your diet, around 90% of cholesterol can be reabsorbed from the intestinal wall space and taken back to the liver. The surplus cholesterol that's returned in this manner to the liver will never be reprocessed and removed again by this organ but rather finds its way into general circulation. Since it is excessive amounts, it accumulates in the blood (hypercholesterolemia) and starts forming deposits along the walls of the arteries. Thickening of the blood and the forming of fatty debris are the basic causes of cardiovascular disease.

High blood cholesterol is reduced through both diet adjustments and regular, extreme stimulation from the liver, among other remedies such as exercise and relaxation.

Good to know

Cholesterol is produced not only from the excess of fatty acids but also from an excessive amount of sugar and proteins.

Cardiovascular Diseases

Cardio diseases (heavy blood or hyperviscosity, high blood pressure, heart attack, heart stroke, etc.) are numerous and vary in their expression, however, they all fundamentally stem from the same root: the accumulation of fatty substances in the blood.

These substances thicken the blood, which slows its rate of circulation.

If they are deposited on the walls of the arteries, they form fatty lumps (atheromas) within the arteries, reducing their size and blocking the passage of blood. When the blood becomes too dense and stagnant, it coagulates. The clot this forms may clog the vessel at the center (coronary attack), in the heart (heart stroke), or elsewhere in the body (embolism).

These excess fatty substances are substances the liver could have prevented from getting into the blood, had it not been overwhelmed by a diet saturated in "poor" fat and sugars.

Revitalizing and detoxifying the liver, therefore, can be an integral part of any treatment for coronary disease.

Do you know?

Thousands of people get blood thinners to fight the thickening of the blood due to liver deficiency and overeating. In America, a billion dollars, annually, is usually spent on prescriptions for anticoagulant medicines.

Hemorrhoids

Hemorrhoids are distensions from the blood veins in the anal region and for that reason a type of varicose veins. These veins connect to the portal vein, which is a large vessel that connects into the liver. When the liver is congested, the movement of the blood that gets to it through the connecting vein is obstructed. It does not travel to the liver as quickly as it should, also it moves in inadequate quantity, so blood starts to accumulate in the portal vein. Among some other consequences, this congested state exerts strain on the anal veins, which forces these to expand and distend.

Added to this pressure is the fact that anal veins contract when someone pushes to evacuate hard stools. This mostly common when there is constipation, a health issue that often accompanies liver deficiency.

Headaches, Migraines

Some headaches and migraines are caused by the distension from the blood vessels in the heart, which creates a painful compression of the surrounding tissues.

This distension from the blood vessels is a defensive reaction to irritating and intense substances being transported with the blood. These substances won't normally make their way into the brain if the liver was functioning well. Several headaches are caused by an inadequacy of the liver in performing its operations.

That is especially true for migraines, which are often accompanied by a sick feeling and vomiting.

Warning

While pain relievers tend to ease headaches momentarily, their long-term effect is usually counterproductive and self-destructive, because by overloading the liver, they decrease its ability to neutralize irritating elements.

Other organs including those far from the liver can suffer

the effects of hepatic deficiency.

Among its other roles, the liver has the responsibility of filtering colloidal wastes which come from foods that are abundant in starch and fat. These types of food are grains and their by-products (for example bread, pasta, and cake), meat, cheese, butter, cream, etc.

Normally the liver removes these wastes from the blood and expels them into the bile to allow them to be removed from the body through stools. When the liver fails to perform this function, the filtration of these substances is prevented and the wastes

stay in the blood and come out of the liver through the hepatic vein.

This enables them to go into general circulation and accumulate in the body's cells terrain. However, your body can defend itself against the accumulation of toxins. If one excretory organ (for example the liver) is not capable of filtering the complete toxin from the body, it will push it to other emunctory organs. After this, the lungs and sebaceous glands take up the duty of eliminating whatever toxins the liver is struggling to filter. When the toxins are too much, these organs will, subsequently, also become worn out and congested. Two common health issues that arise from this condition are the removal of phlegm by the respiratory system and acne.

Respiratory Illnesses (Catarrhal Inflammations)

Wastes that have not been filtered from the blood and the liver make their way into the lungs, bronchial pipes, or sinuses. Their presence in these organs is abnormal as it leads to an inflammation of these mucous membranes, and sometimes a fever. To protect themselves, the membranes secrete a protective mucus that includes the colloidal wastes to be removed. The effect is a heavy removal of phlegm (catarrh), as may be the case during colds, sinusitis, bronchitis, and some forms of asthma.

While there are different types of treatment to provide relief for the respiratory tract, it is only the restoration of the liver to its normal healthy state that will give a lasting solution. As soon as the liver is restored to its normal state, the wastes it now can process won't be able to make their way into the respiratory tract.

Acne

The sebaceous glands in your skin are continuously releasing sebum, an oily substance that lubricates the skin. Sebum contains toxins, the same type as the ones filtered by the liver, so when mentioned above, the sebaceous glands filter some of the wastes the liver is not able to process are caused by being overwhelmed.

These excess toxins are reduced into colloidal wastes by the sebaceous glands, and when they are overwhelmed, they become congested and inflamed which subsequently leads to acne.

Hormonal changes in adolescence tend to be cited as the cause of acne, but liver deficiency plays a major role too. A good liver cleansing is therefore recommended to treat acne.

Colloidal Wastes

These wastes are smooth and viscous, such as phlegm that's expectorated or coughed out and pus that oozes from pimples.

They are the exact opposite of the hard and insoluble crystalline waste that is produced by the body. Types of crystalline waste materials consist of grit-like crystals that accumulate in the important joints or crystals that form kidney stones.

Metabolic Disorders

The accumulation of toxins in the body that happen are caused by a shortcoming in the performance of the liver can also lead to metabolic disorders, such as those linked to sugar or fat.

Hypoglycemia Attacks

Some people are at the mercy of continuous attacks from hypoglycemia (low blood sugar level). They suddenly feel weak and breathless and experience low energy often which is commonly associated with bouts of dizziness and lightheadedness. Most times, they feel stressed and tired. This lack of energy is caused by low sugar in the blood. This causes compelling and repeated cravings for nice foods, such as chocolate, pastries, etc.

Do you know?

Drinking alcohol especially on an empty stomach can prevent your liver from releasing stored glucose into the blood, which can cause hypoglycemia and trigger a repeated desire for more alcoholic drinks or sweet foods.

The main cause of hypoglycemia is the excessive use of bad sugars; however, the liver can also be responsible for the condition. Exercising daily and going about our activities each day helps to "burn up" blood sugar; the content of the sugar in the blood reduces each day but we won't see it. The liver, in its quick and effective manner, instantly corrects the blood sugar level which has fallen too low and restores it to the normal level. This can be done by releasing glucose which has been stored for this purpose through glycogen into the blood.

However, when the liver is completely depleted, the reconversion of glycogen into glucose cannot be properly done. The blood sugar levels, therefore, drop below normal putting the liver in a position where it can do little or nothing.

The perfect solution will be liver detoxification. Once it's been decongested and strengthened, it'll again have the ability to control blood sugar.

An overworked and weak liver is one of the primary causes of obesity. Indeed, fats from the digestive tract go through the liver before they actually reach the cells.

Normally the liver only allows fats that are useful to the body to go into the blood. It transforms the others into cholesterol so that it can be secreted into bile and eliminated through the stool.

Under these circumstances, there is no way you will add unnecessary weight because no extra fat is being sent into the tissues constantly.

On the other hand, when the liver is weak, it cannot transform the excess fats that are not needed by your body into cholesterol, or even if it will do this, it will only be in small quantities.

The excess fats stay in the blood and enter the tissues. This kind of buildup will be proportionate to the level of excess fat the liver cannot cope with and how large the fat substance from the individual's diet plan is.

The liver is an excellent regulator of fats. This describes why diet programs are

not always as effective as they should be.

When eating restrictions decrease the intake of body fat that the liver should treat, they raise the level of fats the tissues to be burned up and used, among other activities, to provide energy. However, going on a diet does not instantly enhance the ability of a weak and overworked liver to take care of these released excess fats.

Because of this it often happens that the individual following the diet plan might have difficulty sticking to it but has little success as the liver isn't complying. It is not able to get rid of the excess fats.

All diets designed for weight reduction should therefore end up being with a good plan for liver detoxification to assist it in its job of managing excess fat.

The Disease Fighting Capability

The deficiencies of the liver can be so pronounced that the number of unfiltered toxins it allows to feed will eventually disrupt it's disease fighting ability. This is the foundation of several problems and illnesses.

Cancer

Nearly all cancers are caused by toxins that alter the genetic code of the cells in a harmful way. Tissues then begin to multiply in a disorganized way and then form tumors. The part of toxins responsible for the proliferation of malignancies has led to them being called carcinogenic or mutagenic substances.

The most common are:

- Excessive alcohol

- Arsenic and cyanide (from cigarettes)

- Methylxanthine from coffee, tea, cola beverages, and cocoa

- Tars in grilled food (and besides roasted coffee beans)

- Benzo[the]pyrene found in smoked foods (meat, fish)

- Certain chemical substance food additives

- Mycotoxins from the molds that develop on coffee beans and grains not stored properly.

- Nitrosamines (nitrates) excessive amounts found in water in certain areas, also in some meals (particularly processed meats) and cosmetics.

- Heavy metals from pollution

- Certain medications

This list is surprisingly like the set of harmful substances in the liver's job description. A liver that functions effectively is one of the fundamental components of fighting cancer since it can neutralize the mutagenic substances that trigger the formation of cancerous tumors. Its action isn't just preventive; it is also healing.

Actually, its effective detoxifying abilities free of charge the mobile terrain of overloads of toxins that support the formation of tumors.

The truth that the liver is an important organ in the fight against cancer has been established by some researchers, but that is not enough.

Autoimmune Diseases

In these increasingly common diseases (polyarthritis, lupus erythematosus, etc.), the disease-fighting ability destroys the tissues in your body it is meant to protect. What can cause this?

Whenever a person eats large portions of food containing chemical additives, contaminants, and several other toxins, these substances accumulate in the tissues, i.e. inside the tissue of your skin, the muscle tissues, the skeleton, etc. Because they are now filled with destructive materials, the immune system no longer sees these cells' material as normal tissues forming sections of the body but as invasive and dangerous cells. After that, it turns against them and tries to eliminate them.

The best treatment for these diseases requires restoring the liver to its normal state that prevents the tissues from collecting a lot of toxic substances. The disease-fighting ability protects the body by destroying whatever attacks it. The liver stops harmful chemicals from entering farther into the body. This way a healthy liver protects the disease-fighting ability. So it becomes as obvious as the" Liver Doctor" Sandra Cabot explains, "Diseases from the disease-fighting ability are always frustrated by the exact thing that stresses the liver or overwhelms it," This is where it begins in the body.

Allergies

An allergic attack is the disease-fighting ability to release an exaggerated histamine response to a substance that is not actually posing any threat to your body.

 This substance is not a germ or even something toxic but an otherwise inoffensive substance such as an airborne irritant (pollen, dust), some sort of food (fermented meals, alcohol, cheese, etc.), or insect venom. People who are prone to allergies generally metabolize histamine poorly and also have trouble using and eliminating it.

How does an allergen enter the body? An allergen can enter either through the mouth, pores, and skin, or lungs. The disease-fighting ability identifies it as potentially dangerous and mobilizes antibodies to attack it. The antibodies trigger the discharge of histamine (inflammatory chemical substances) to result in the body's immune system.

However, histamine also increases inflammation, so once it has been used for defense purposes, it should be neutralized and eliminated. This technique can take place directly in the tissue or within the heart but can be a function performed by the liver.

When the histamine isn't neutralized and removed, it remains stagnant in the tissues and puts the body in a pre-inflammatory and hyperreactive condition.

Symptoms of this may include congestion, rash, shortness of breath, coughing, etc.

The hyperreactivity of the immune system can also be caused by the attack and irritation of the body by harmful toxins that the liver should neutralize and eliminate.

Therefore, good detoxification of the liver is the right treatment when coping with any kind of allergy, whether it's hay fever, bronchial asthma, hives, rash, angioedema (Quincke's edema), or an allergy affecting the digestive tract.

Chapter 8

Dietary Reform

Since the liver is the first organ to get all substances that have been prepared by digestion, its strength and resistance are closely reliant on what we eat.

You can consider these three aspects that pertain to diet about the liver:

- Foods to eliminate from our diet plan. Some foods overwhelm the liver, attack it, or even force it to overwork. It is essential to identify these types of food so we can exclude them from our daily diet.

- The diet plan is beneficial to the liver. We are to feed ourselves in a way that is adapted towards the liver's abilities. This is the diet we have to follow to aid and strengthen this body organ.

- The detoxifying diet plan. A restrictive diet, limited by a set time frame, will provide relief to the liver and help it to cleanse itself of all toxins that have already been congesting it.

Foods To Remove

Some foods place a heavy need on the liver without

offering many benefits to the body, and can even be harmful. The liver exhausts itself changing and neutralizing the toxins these types of foods bring into the body. Ultimately its capabilities turn out to be reduced and weakened until it can no longer perform its work effectively.

Foods to eliminate from your diet plan include:

- Hydrogenated margarine (filled with saturated essential fatty acids which are now often called trans fats)
- Heat-pressed oils
- Chilly cuts and sausages
- Smoked foods (fish and meat)
- Foods with a high sugar content
- Food cooked inside butter
- Fried foods
- Chips
- Alcohol
- Coffee and dark tea
- Food items containing additives

Bad Fats

Bad fat requires the exertion of most of the liver's strength in the digestion process, which reduces the strength it has reserved for detoxification. Also, excess fatty acids gather in the liver and disrupt its operations (the symptoms of the congested fatty liver).

Some people believe they're doing their livers a huge favor by eliminating the use of any kind of fat, whether it is of animal or veggie origin. However, this is not the case.

If you don't include fat in what you eat, your gallbladder won't be able to store the bile it secretes into the digestive system. The bile will remain stagnant in your gallbladder, where it will thicken and pose a great risk of forming gallstones. Furthermore, because the muscle tissue in the gallbladder is no longer working as much as it should, they'll lose their firmness, and this can weaken the body organ.

The assimilation of liposoluble (soluble in fatty substances) vitamins such as vitamins D, E, and F (omega-3 and omega-6) may also be compromised.

On the other hand, because these vitamins are found in fatty foods that this person is not any longer eating since they are missing from the dietary plan and whatever requirements they fulfill in the body will go unmet. In the same way, these vitamins require bile to be assimilated, the bile that the body lacks because no demand has been placed on the gallbladder so that they will even now not meet up with the body's requirements.

Quite simply, while it is essential to remove bad fats, the body needs healthy fats to be able to function properly.

An Ailing Liver and Fats

A person's diet plans should contain low animal fats because they are saturated in fatty acids, and this is however based on how sick or weak the liver is.

Fats from herb sources (virgin cold-pressed natural oils) and oleaginous nut products and seed products are rich in unsaturated fatty acids. The liver can tolerate these kinds of fats more easily, but caution should be taken and the quantities ought to be adapted based on the individual's capacity.

Excessive White-colored Sugars and Sweets

Eating excessive levels of sweets, especially those made out of white sugars, is bad for the liver, as all unneeded sugar is usually transformed into body fat and cholesterol that stagnates within the liver and blood.

Alcohol, Food Chemicals, and Smoked Foods

These kinds of foods exhaust the liver since it is the liver's responsibility to neutralize the toxins they contain.

Tobacco, Medicines, and Medications

These substances are not foods themselves, however, they are substances that people ingest and are bad for the liver.

Enemies of the Liver

- **Excessive Alcohol**: 95% of the alcohol ingested by your body is neutralized by the liver.

- **Smokes**: They contain many toxins (pure nicotine, arsenic, formaldehyde, etc.).

- **Medications**: Most medications are usually damaging to liver cells, especially analgesics, bodily hormones, antibiotics, and anti-inflammatories; these medicines should only be used when they are necessary.

- **Medications**: heroin, cocaine, etc.

- **Chemical pollutants**: Food chemicals, agricultural chemicals, heavy metals from air pollution, solvents, paints, etc.

- **Overeating generally**: It stresses the liver.

- **Excessive fat in the diet plan**: greasy meats, chilly cuts, pâtés, sausages, deep-fried foods, foods sautéed in butter, hydrogenated margarine.

- **White sugar and nice foods**: All extra sugar ingested by your body will undoubtedly be converted into fat.

- **Smoked foods**: Fish, meats.

The Liver-Friendly Diet

The diet that is good for the liver is not just one that will not overwork the liver during digestion but will also not produce toxins that the organ cannot easily neutralize and eliminate. Another quality of this diet plan is that it supplies the liver with much nutrition that helps to optimize its functionality.

Foods that are in this section of a liver-friendly diet plan are split into three groups. Each is intrinsically beneficial, however, not in the same measure. Some can be consumed regularly, whereas others should be consumed in more moderate amounts because they exert a lot of pressure on the liver. Also, there are a few that needs to be eaten in restricted measures due to the work they place on the liver. They, however, are part of the diet plan since they supply essential nutrients, such as proteins to the body and the liver.

Eat As You Desire

- Natural and cooked vegetables
- Raw fruits
- Germinated grains
- Water and plant tea
- Unsweetened fruits and vegetable juices
- Natural herbs and spices (excluding chili pepper flakes)

Eat-In Moderation

- Nuts
- Little seeds: sunflower, flax, pumpkin along with other squash
- Starches: potatoes, grain, chestnuts
- Whole grains
- Bread, crackers, and pasta created from whole-grain flour

Eat-In Small Quantities

- Meat

- Fish

- Dairy products

- Eggs

- Cold-pressed plant oils

- Sweeteners: honey, maple syrup, pear, and other fruits syrups without added sugar or even fructose

It is better to prioritize fruits & vegetables that are grown naturally, in addition to milk products, eggs, and meat of free-range animals that have been given a natural diet plan, as these types of food are free from toxic chemicals (herbicides, pesticides, growth hormones, antibiotics) and their ingestion will undoubtedly be gentler on the liver, and also to the environment. Choose whole food items as much as possible, instead of processed foods, since they supply more of the nutrients the liver requires.

Also, it is important to make "lighting," which is to state with a minimum of body fat (boiled, steamed, baked).

The Detoxifying Diet

Removing foods that can damage the liver from the diet plan and adopting one that will nourish the organ is necessary to allow the liver to recover its power and also restore its health in a gradual process. This repair will take some time, however, to speed up the detoxification of the liver, it is possible to follow a more restrictive diet plan.

Whenever we make fewer demands on the liver during the digestive process, it can make use of its strength to eliminate toxins that have accumulated in it. Instead of dealing with arriving toxins, it must only cope with congested residue. This significantly accelerates the detoxification process.

There are different types of the restrictive diet of any nature. A diet is said to be restrictive when someone eats intentionally less than what he or she usually eats.

The more restrictive the diet is, the faster the results, however, it can be hard to stick to this diet plan since it involves both physical and psychological deprivation.

Guidelines

A balanced diet includes:

⅔ salads and vegetables

⅓ starches and proteins

How It Works

The diet I'm suggesting here is moderately restrictive and should be able to fit anyone's need. It is simply eating nothing but fruit and veggies for a period of one to three days. The veggies can be consumed raw, prepared, or juiced. Homemade veggie soups are another option. Prepared vegetables should be steamed, boiled, or baked (without essential oil). Fruits can also be consumed raw, cooked, or juiced. No sugar should be added to these, but juices could be diluted with water if you like.

The digestion break allows the liver to cleanse itself of toxins. If at the end of the first day of the diet, you are feeling great, filled with energy and strength with no indicators of exhaustion, you should continue for another day and even the next.

Chapter 9

What foods protect the Liver?

The liver is responsible for breaking down food, building glucose, and detoxifying the body. It also stores nutrition and produces bile, which is necessary to break down and absorb the nutrients in food. There are lots of foods and beverages that an individual can consume to help protect the liver.

The health of the liver is essential for general health. Liver dysfunction can cause liver illness, metabolic disorder, and type 2 diabetes.

While it can be impossible to control all possibilities of liver disease, eating healthily can help to protect the health of the liver.

In this chapter, we will discuss the best foods to eat to protect the health of the liver, their benefits, and some foods to avoid.

Best foods and beverages for Liver health

Some of the best foods and beverages that help to protect

the health of the liver include:

Coffee

A 2013 study that was published in the Liver International journal shows that more than 50% of Americans drink coffee every day.

Coffee is good for the liver, especially since it protects against diseases such as fatty liver conditions.

The review also notes that everyday coffee intake can help reduce the threat of chronic liver disease. It can also protect the liver from injuries like liver cancer.

A 2014 research that appeared in the Journal of Clinical Gastroenterology shows that the protective effects of coffee are because of how it affects liver enzymes.

Coffee, in reviews, appears to reduce fat buildup in the liver. It also raises protective antioxidants in the liver. Compounds in coffee also help liver enzymes rid your body of cancer-causing substances.

Oatmeal

Eating oatmeal is an easy way to include fiber in the dietary plan. Fiber is an essential food to aid digestion, and the exact materials in oats are especially ideal for the liver. Oats and oatmeal are high in substances called beta-glucans.

In a 2017 research in the International Journal of Molecular Sciences reviews, beta-glucans have become biologically mixed up in the body. They help in improving the disease-fighting ability of the body and prevent inflammation, and they are also specifically useful in the fight against diabetes and obesity.

The review also notes that beta-glucans from oats can help to reduce the quantity of fat stored in the liver in bits, and can also help to protect the liver. However, more clinical studies are needed to approve this claim.

People who want to include oats or oatmeal in their diet plan should look for whole oats or steel-cut oats, instead of prepackaged oatmeal. Prepackaged oatmeal may contain fillers such as flour or sugar, which may not be good for the body.

Green tea

A 2015 study in the World Journal of Gastroenterology says that green tea extract can help to reduce overall body fat, fight oxidative tension, and reduce some other signs of non-alcoholic fatty liver illness (NAFLD).

You should note that green tea can be better than components, as some ingredients may harm the liver instead of healing it.

The study notes that there are still no specific instructions on whether those with this condition should take tea or tea extracts, however, the road to a healthy liver is promising.

Garlic

Adding garlic clove to the dietary plan can also help to stimulate the liver. A 2016 research that was published in the Advanced Biomedical Study journal notes that eating garlic clove reduces body weight and fats in people who have NAFLD, without changing the physical features. This is advantageous, as being obese contributes to

NAFLD.

Berries

Many dark berries, such as blueberries, raspberries, and cranberries, contain antioxidants called polyphenols, which might help to protect the liver from damage.

As a report of the World Journal of Gastroenterology suggests, feeding on berries regularly helps to stimulate the disease-fighting ability of the liver.

Grapes

A study from the World Journal of Gastroenterology reports that grapes, grape juice, and grape seeds are rich in antioxidants that can help the liver to reduce inflammation and prevent liver damage.

Eating whole seeded grapes is a simple way to include these substances in your dietary plan. A grape seed draws-out supplement can also provide antioxidants.

Grapefruit

The World Journal of Gastroenterology study also mentions grapefruit as helpful food. Grapefruit consists of two main antioxidants: naringin and naringenin. These can help protect the liver from injuries by reducing swelling and protecting the liver tissues.

The compounds can also reduce fat buildup in the liver and aid the enzymes that remove fats. This makes grapefruit a useful diet in the fight against NAFLD.

Prickly pear

The fruit and juice from the prickly pear are also good for liver health. The world journal of Gastroenterology research suggests that substances in the fruits can help to protect the organ.

Most research focus on the extracts from the fruits, however, researches that concentrate on fruits and juice is also important.

Plant foods generally

A 2015 research that was published in the Evidence-based Complementary and Option Medicine journal states a large number of herb foods that are ideal for the liver. They include:

- Avocado
- Banana
- Barley
- beets and beet juice
- broccoli
- brown rice
- carrots
- fig
- greens such as kale and collards
- lemon
- papaya
- watermelon

People should eat this kind of foods in a complete and balanced diet plan.

Fatty fish

In a report by the World Journal of Gastroenterology, eating fatty seafood and seafood oil supplements can help to decrease the effects of conditions like NAFLD.

Fatty fish is rich in omega-3 essential fatty acids, which is the fat that reduces inflammation. This fat is especially helpful in the liver because they prevent the accumulation of excess body fat and keep maintaining enzyme levels in the liver.

The analysis recommends taking oily fish several times every week. If it's not easy to include fatty fish such as herring or salmon in the diet plan, try going for a daily fish essential oil supplement.

Nuts

The same study says that eating nuts is another easy way to keep the liver healthy prevent NAFLD. Nuts contain unsaturated essential fatty acids, vitamin e antioxidants, and antioxidants. These substances can fight against NAFLD, and also reduce irritation and oxidative tension. Eating a small number of nuts, such as walnuts or almonds, every day can sustain the liver's health. You should be careful not to eat too much of it because nuts contain calories.

Olive oil

Eating an excessive amount of fat isn't good for the liver, however, some levels of fats can help it. Based on the World Journal of Gastroenterology study, adding essential olive oil to the dietary plan can reduce oxidative stress and improve the performance of the liver. This is due to the high content of unsaturated fatty acids in the oil.

Chapter 10

Detoxing Plant-Based Recipes Good for Your Liver

Have you tried a detox system? Drinking lemon and cayenne juice most of the time, feeling awful, and losing weight that somehow magically reappeared? It seems that we have all tried one kind of detoxification or another. Maybe it made you feel better for a while, but then the satisfaction you get from the treatment disappears all too soon.

Have made out time to figure what meals are healthy for your liver? What about the kidneys? Perhaps you have thought about your lymphatic system that contains a huge selection of lymph nodes lately? Many of these body parts are usually effective in detoxing. The spleen "detects possibly dangerous bacteria, infections, or some other microorganisms in the blood," the liver removes "toxins from the body through urine or stool" and bile, as well as the kidneys "filtrate 120 to 150 quarts of blood each day and create one or two quarts of urine" which consists of toxins along with other waste.

Having said that, even though your body can do the cleansing jobs alone, it is always a good idea to get the perfect plant-based foods that assist the organs that are responsible for ridding the body of toxins. Luckily, there's a complete list of plant-based food to help you to accomplish this!

Cold Brew Snow Cream Cold Brew Glaciers Cream

Coffee not only gives you a little pick and choose me personally up but it's also ideal for the liver! Coffee "protects against problems like a fatty liver disease" and can "reduce the risk of a chronic liver disease." This Chilly Brew Ice Lotion recipe by Deena Jalal is a superb treat that may furthermore infuse you with a wholesome dosage of liver-protecting espresso!

This recipe uses your preferred real, cold-brewed coffee, concentrated to infuse extra flavor and reduce iciness. Therefore, use coffee you'll beverage- it's the celebrity of the display. If you're not a coffee ice lotion fan, this recipe might just switch your mind.

Ingredients

1 /3 mug (60 g) medium-ground coffees

2 1/2 mugs (600 ml) all-natural canned coconut milk

1/4 cup (50 g) organic unrefined cane sugar

1/4 cup (60 ml) agave

1 tablespoon (15 ml) real vanilla extract

Pinch of salt

Preparation

- In a dish, combine the coffee grounds and coconut milk. Protect this combination and stick it in the fridge to steep overnight, at the very least 12 hrs. or more.

- As soon as it's steeped, work with a fine-mesh strainer to eliminate the grounds from your coconut dairy. If you discover your coconut whole milk has divided and there's a coating of cream at the top, mix it and allow milk warm plenty to homogenize before straining it. Discard the lands.

- Work with a high-speed or immersion blender to combine the coconut dairy coffee, sugars, agave, vanilla, and Salt. Add the blend for your snow cream producer and churn is based on the manufacturer's guidelines. Most machines get 10 to quarter-hour with regards to the temperature from the mix, so when it's completed it should appear to be soft serve.

- As soon as it's churned, move the ice lotion to a big freezer-safe container, clean the very best, and cover-up it firmly. Freeze the completed ice lotion for at the very least 5 to 6 hrs, or until it is firm. Shop this ice lotion in the refrigerator in a covered container for 1 week.

Kale Salad Stability Bowl

Kale is a champ dark leafy natural containing a "wide range of nutritional vitamins, fibers, and nutrients," in addition to kidney-protecting "substances such as antioxidants." This Kale Salad Stability Bowl recipe by Crissy Cavanaugh also includes fiber-rich nice potatoes, coffee beans, and quinoa, which can help to protect your liver.

Kale Salad Stability Bowl with dark coffee beans, harissa roasted lovely potatoes, and special tahini dressing for any balanced dinner in a bowl!

Serves 2

Cooking Time 30mins

Ingredients

For that Roasted Sweet Potatoes:

1 large sugary potato, peeled and cubed (~1/2 mugs)

A drizzle of oil

1/2 teaspoon powdered harissa

Salt to taste

For your Sweet Tahini Dressing:

1/2 cup tahini

1/2 cup water

2 tablespoons Bragg's proteins (or tamari/soy sauce)

2 tablespoons agave (or maple syrup)

2 tablespoons toasted sesame seed oil

1 tablespoon apple cider vinegar

1 tablespoon miso paste

For the Salad:

3 mugs of kale, destemmed and chopped

a drizzle of oil

Salt to taste

1 cup cooked dark beans (or canned beans, rinsed and drained)

1/2 cup prepared quinoa (optional)

2 tablespoons of dried fruits such as cranberries or raisins

Preparation

For that Roasted Sweet Potatoes:

- Preheat oven to 350°F. Toss cubed nice potatoes having a drizzle of essential olive oil, switch to a cooking sheet, and sprinkle with powdered harissa and salt. Bake for 20-30 moments or until sensitive when pierced with a fork.

For your Sweet Tahini Dressing:

- Add all the ingredients to a higher rate blender and mix until it is well blended and emulsified.

At the Salad:

- In a dish, drizzle kale with essential olive oil and put in a dash of sea salt. Use fingers to therapeutic massage kale until nicely coated with essential oil.

- Add coffee beans, massaged kale, and roasted lovely potatoes to some dish. Toss in prepared quinoa and some dried-out cranberries if preferred.

- Dress it up and enjoy!

White Chocolates Lemon Snacks Truffles

Citrus is one of the foods that aid a wholesome lymphatic system because they contain "powerful enzymes, and Supplement C, that assist your body and preserve digestion streaming." This White Colored Chocolate Lemon Snacks Truffles recipe by Kat Condon is the perfect solution to get you an everyday dose of citrus in an ideal snack-sized meal!

The perfect special and salty treat, these white chocolate lemon popcorn truffles are an ode to spring! It'll satisfy your sugary tooth as well as your craving for crunchy snack foods without being overweight. The snacks themselves are durable but not excessively crisp, which gives it an extremely delicious "truffle" middle.

Serves 18-20

Ingredients

4 cups popcorn

1/4 cup shredded, unsweetened coconut

1/2 cup coconut oil, soft

1/4 cup maple syrup

1 bag vegan whitened chocolate chips or create your own

1 lemon, zested

More lemon zest, for topping

Preparation

- Line a cooking sheet with parchment or polished paper. Reserve.

- Toss snacks and coconut in a large dish.

- Cream collectively the coconut essential oil and maple syrup until clean. Pour over snacks mixture, then use your fingers, toss to coating well. Put the mix inside the fridge for ten minutes to solidify.

- Using a spoonful at a time, press the popcorn mixture together in your hands until it forms a ball. It's okay if popcorn gets crushed. Wet hands to make handling easier. Place popcorn balls into the baking sheet.

- Once all the popcorns have been formed into balls, put in the freezer for five minutes.

- While snacks are chilling, melt your white chocolate chips. Include lemon zest, which stirs until smooth, and reserve for a couple of minutes to cool. If chocolate will be hot, it will melt the coconut oil and the snacks balls will break apart.

- Taking it separately, drop the popcorn balls into the whitened chocolate. Move around such that it will be fully coated, after that put it back on the cooking sheet. Sprinkle with additional lemon zest. Do it again with the remaining snacks until all have already been coated in whitened chocolate. Store in the fridge until you're ready to eat.

Spelt-Flax Crackers with Sunflower Seed Pate

How do seed products help to keep your cleansing organs and techniques running smoothly? Works out these teeny small morsels carry much weight of magnesium - which helps the nervous program - and healthful fat - which lubricate your body and strengthen your lymph circulation! This Spelt-Flax Cracker with Sunflower Seed Pate recipe by Courtney Western not only supplies a healthy dose of sunflowers, but it's also a good way to obtain flax.

These homemade crackers have an ideal crunch. The pate will be creamy, with a level of tanginess. Use these crackers and pate alongside any distribution, like hummus or cashew cheese, being an appetizer at events and they'll be considered a nice dish.

Ingredients

For that Spelt and Flax Crackers:

1/2 cup, plus 1 tablespoon of flour

1/2 cup flax meal

1 teaspoon cooking powder

1/4 teaspoon okay grain ocean salt

2 teaspoons natural sugar

3 tablespoons of oil

3 tablespoons water

For your Lemon Dill Sunflower Pate:

1 cup natural sunflower kernels, soaked for at the very least 6 hours

2-3 tablespoons oil

2 tablespoons new dill

1 tablespoon refreshing lemon juice

1/8 teaspoon roasted garlic powder

The pinch of sea salt

Preparation

To help make the Crackers:

- Preheat your oven to 400°F. Use either a silicon baking sheet or a sheet of parchment prepared (you'll move the cracker dough from this before putting it on your sheet skillet).

- Whisk the dry components together until it is smooth. Create a nicely in the center, then add water and oil. Mix with a spatula or wood spoon before dough all fits in place. Dust the hands with some flour, after that knead the dough several times until it is smooth.

- Gently dust your baking sheet. Place the dough on the sheet and move it out having a moving pin until it is about 1/16-in. thick, making certain to keep this for the sheet.

- Using a pastry or pizza cutter, slice the dough into squares, then work with a fork to prick the crackers. Move the sheet for your cooking sheet and bake the crackers for 8-12 mins until they're golden and sharp at the sides.

- Remove through the oven and determine if you want to re-cut the crackers (the dough should distance itself since it bakes, causing this to be unnecessary). Cool for 10 minutes in the sheet, and then transfer to the rack to cool completely.

To help make the Pate:

- Soak the sunflower seed products. Put them in a medium-sized dish, cover up them with drinking water, and allow them to soak right away or for at least 6-8 hours. Drain and wash them before making use of them.

- In a food processor or high-speed blender, course of action the ingredients until thick, creamy paste forms. After the pate will be solid and creamy, flavor it, and change for seasoning. Eat immediately with the spelled and flax crackers or anyone of your choice.

Beet 'n' Berry Overnight Cauliflower Oats

Oatmeal is a superb way to start the day off, and it also "could be especially ideal for the liver" because of beta-glucans, which "lessen the quantity of fat stored in the liver." This Beet 'n' Berry Overnight Cauliflower Oats recipe by Tara Sunlight also includes plenty of berries, which certainly are excellent antioxidant-rich support meals for that kidney as well as the lymphatic system.

These beet & berry overnight oats will be the ideal breakfast for hectic mornings. They are very healthy and tasty and the color is gorgeous! Make them a night before and you can simply get them and proceed each day! Or scoop them into a dish and enjoy a good breakfast and never have to worry about rendering it.

Ingredients

1/3 cup gluten-free old-fashioned rolled oats

1/2 cup unsweetened almond or nut-free milk

1/2 cup iced raspberries

1/2 cup iced cauliflower rice (steamed-then-frozen if

necessary for better digestion)

2 tablespoons simple homemade coconut yogurt

one to two 2 tablespoons vegan vanilla proteins powder

1 tablespoon chia seeds

1 tablespoon red beet crystals

1 teaspoon gelatinized maca natural powder (optionally available)

1/2 teaspoon reishi, lion's mane, or 6 mushroom blend natural powder (optional)

monk fruit sweetener or any sweetener of your choice, adjusted to taste

optionally available toppings: coconut chips (matcha-flavored kinds right here), granola, grapes, new or iced berries, bee pollen, or toppings of preference

Preparation

- Put all the components (excluding toppings) right in a dish or single-serving mason jar(s) and blend well to mix. Sweeten to flavor.
- Cover up and refrigerate immediately, or for at least 6 hours.

- Each day, stir and serve chilled or heat if desired. Add toppings and enjoy!

Spinach Artichoke Quesadillas

More dark leafy greens for the kidney! Plus, spinach supplies an entire dose of metal together with those antioxidants. This Spinach Artichokes Quesadillas recipe by Rene Barker is ideal for an instant and healthy treat chock filled with healthy fat, nutritional vitamins, and minerals!

Artichoke drop is hot, cheesy, and comforting. Imagine if you place those tastes and feelings into a tortilla? Growth, that is what these quesadillas are usually! They are ooey, gooey, and very delicious.

Serves 2-4

Cooking Time 10

Ingredients

1/2 teaspoon oil

1 garlic clove diced

6 ounces marinated artichoke hearts diced

3 cups of baby spinach

4 ounces of vegan cream cheese

2 tablespoons of vegan mayonnaise

Salt and pepper to taste

Crimson pepper flakes (optional)

2 large flour tortillas

Preparation

- Heat oil in a skillet over a low fire. Add the garlic clove and sauté for a minute, stirring frequently. Add artichoke hearts and 2 glasses of baby spinach. Stir to mix and cook until spinach starts to wilt.

- Add lotion cheese, mayo, salt, pepper, and red pepper flakes to skillet and stir to mix. Warm through and reserve.

- Put a big non-stick skillet on the range over medium-high temperature. Put 1 tortilla in the skillet and fill up with 1/2 of the spinach artichoke combination and another 1/2 mug of baby spinach – ensuring to blend 1/2 of the tortilla.

- Fold tortilla in two and prepare until the bottom starts to brownish (approx. 2 minutes). Stir and cook until the part is brown as well. Remove from the pan and repeat the process with the remaining ingredients.

- Slice and enjoy.

Miracle Bread

While sunflower seed products are perfect for boosting lymph wellness, hemp seed products are directly on their coattails! This Wonder Bread recipe by Natalie Yonan is packed with hemp seed products, pumpkin seed products, chia seed products, and flax seed products, all bundled as well as coconut essential oil, maple syrup, and psyllium husk natural powder.

Say hello to the prettiest bread around! Vegan, gluten-free, and deliciously tasty!

Calories 2591

Ingredients

For the Dry Ingredients:

1/2 cups gluten-free rolled oats

1 cup pumpkin seeds

1 cup raw turned on nuts

1/3 cup hemp seeds

1 teaspoon salt

2 1/2 tablespoons chia seeds

3 tablespoons psyllium husks powder

1/4 cup flax seeds

For the Wet Ingredients:

3 tablespoons melted coconut oil

2 1/2 tablespoons maple syrup

1/2 cups cold to warm water

Preparation

- Add all the dry ingredients to in big dish and mix gently.
- Add the wet ingredients after the dry ones ingredients and mix well.
- Pour the mixture into a parchment-lined 11x5 loaf skillet. It should be tightly packed!
- Cover and allow it to be there for at least two hours.
- Preheat oven to 375 F. Bake for 20 mins. Take out from the stove. Flip a loaf of bread over and place it on the cooking rack and bake for another thirty

minutes.

- Allow the bread to be properly baked before cutting it. Enjoy!

Baked Apples

Apples are not only great to fulfill a raging nice tooth, but they also have a soluble fiber called pectin, which "can help reduce quite a few risks related to kidney harm, such as high blood sugar levels and cholesterol amounts." This Baked apple recipe by Gabriela Lupu is incredibly simple yet tasty! With a wholesome dose of excess fat from coconut oil and walnuts, lymphatic program boosting lemon fruit juice, and a little bit of inflammation-reducing cinnamon, they are an ideal dessert for a healthy household.

This is the smell of Christmas in your kitchen. These cooked apples are simple and completely delicious. Use apples that are ripe if you want the cooked apples to come out well.

Cooking Time 40

Ingredients

4 -6 apples

1 teaspoon cinnamon

1/2 cup walnuts

2 tablespoons coconut oil

3 tablespoons maple syrup

1 tablespoon lemon juice

Preparation

- Change the oven to 400°F. With a little spoon, scoop out the insides and seed from each apple around the bottom (usually do not move complete apple). Arrange apples, cavity part up, inside a cup, or ceramic cooking tray. I used my banana loaf cooking tray.
- In a dish blend the cinnamon, coconut oil, honey, walnuts, and lemon juice.
- Fill up each cavity using the walnut combination. Sprinkle walnut blend together with the apples.
- Bake the apples 30 to 40 for a few minutes or and soon you like how sensitive they're. Rotate the cooking tray halfway with the baking.

- Serve it warm, as simple as it is, or become inspired and add vanilla ice gel or the best: sour cherry jam. Sour and nice tastes heavenly.

Homemade Golden Flax Seed Milk

This Homemade Golden Flax Seed Dairy recipe by Wendy Irene has a few wonderful plant-based things that will also increase your lymphatic system including high fiber flax seeds, hemp seeds, and cinnamon.

Making your alternative milk in the home is simple and satisfying! For this recipe, use 1 fantastic flax seed because they're thought to have a milder taste, but brown works just fine as well. The times and vanilla have sweetness towards the recipe that I'd not recommend missing. Cinnamon is optionally available, the flax dairy tastes good without it, but if you're a big lover of cinnamon because of its additional nutrients and taste, go on and test it out.

Calories 55

Serves 4

Ingredients

6 mugs filtered water

1/4 cup golden flax seeds

4 dates, pitted

2 teaspoons pure vanilla extract

1/4 teaspoon cinnamon (optional - if you want the taste of cinnamon in your drinks)

Preparation

- Add water and flaxseed products to some high-speed blender. Mix on higher for a minute

- Strain flax whole milk with a nut dairy handbag into a dish, or through a colander lined with cheesecloth folded over once or twice. It is beneficial to make use of tongs or the hands to press and coax the flax whole milk through the handbag. (*Suggestion - When the handbag becomes overly blocked and isn't draining, simply put the rest of the flax dairy back to the blender, wash nut whole milk handbag off to unclog it, and add the remaining milk through the handbag again.)

- Wash flax seed items from the blender, and put the strained flax dairy back to the blender mixed with the pitted dates, real vanilla draw out, and cinnamon when you are using it.

- Blend on high for a moment.
- Skim coating of foam off the very best from the flax milk.
- Store in the refrigerator, and mix or shake before serving.

The 3-Component Berry Cereal

Berries, especially blackberries including "blueberries, raspberries, and cranberries" are rich with "antioxidants called polyphenols, which can help to protect the liver from harm." Add spice to your regular breakfast with this particular 3-Component Berry Cereal recipe by Sara Grandominico, and a rocking solution to obtain that extra dietary fiber to help keep you healthy for long!

Everyone loves it because it brings back that nostalgia of childhood and getting up on the Saturday early morning with the weekend stretched out before you and immediately downing a plate of genuine sugar. This vegan three-ingredient berry cereal is here now to rectify that sugar crash! This breakfast brings back those warm, fuzzy childhood cereal memories and it's healthy and plant-based. It's made out of just three simple ingredients and it'll fill you up.

Serves 3 cups

Cooking Time 30

Ingredients

3 cups gluten-free wholegrain rolled oats, floor into flour

1 cup day paste (about 16 Medjool schedules combined with 1 cup warm water)

1/2 cups refreshing berries, blended

Preparation

- Preheat the oven to 350°F.
- Mix the oats until they look like flour.
- Measure 1 glass of oat flour into 3 separate bowls.
- Make the date paste, then measure out 1/3 mug of paste into each one of the 3 bowls.
- Puree 1/2 glass of berries, and place into one bowl. Repeat with the rest of the berries and enhance the remaining dishes of batter.
- Stir to mix each plate of batter until thoroughly mixed.
- Get about 3 teaspoons of batter, roll into a golf ball,

and put on the lined cooking sheet. Do it again until all the batters are on the baking sheet.

- Bake the cereal for thirty minutes.
- Allow the cereal to cool and sit out for approximately 2 hours. That is when it gets crunchy!

Tofu Scramble and Collard Greens

Dark leafy greens, such as collard greens, are not only ideal for your kidney health but, are also among the top plant-based products in reducing inflammation. Begin or end your day with this particular Tofu Scramble and Collard Greens recipe by Alex Wolfe. This recipe is filled with protein, antioxidants, healthful excess fat, and inflammation-fighting agents.

Cooking Time 20

Ingredients

1/2 case of cut Collard Greens from Investor Joe's

1 small tomato

1/2 stop of extra Company Tofu

1 tablespoon of turmeric

pinch of salt

1 medium-sized yellowish bell pepper, chopped

half a crimson onion, sliced in rings

two cloves of garlic clove, minced

1/4 leek, chopped in 1/4" rings

2 shakes of Paprika

Olive oil

Preparation

- First, get a large soup pot and pour in a few olive oils. Add the onion, and leeks and sautee over medium-high warmth for about five minutes or before onions turn a little bit translucent. Halfway through add the garlic clove. After, add the bell peppers and prepare for another three minutes, stirring frequently to be sure everything will be coated in a lot of oil and isn't sticking to the bottom of the pot. Add whatever spices you prefer! Lastly, add those collards in the pot and toss (either with a wooden spoon or some tongs) until nicely integrated. Cook before greens is wilted, as pictured above.

- Meanwhile, in a little frying pan put in a bit of olive

oil to coat the bottom. Get the tofu and crumble with your fingertips until it becomes a little pebble size (you can't do that wrong, so simply get in there and become brave). Add the turmeric and Salt (experiment using the turmeric until it suits your taste. Add the tomatoes. Cook under medium-high temperature until somewhat crispy, about 7 moments. Use a slim metallic spatula to scrape the tofu that sticks to the bottom part of the skillet (this, if you ask me, maybe the yummiest component).

Basic Homemade Pumpkin Seed Butter

Think it is possible to only create plant-based butter from nut products? Turns out seed products are filled with healthful fatty natural oils that, when mixed, become a very tasty, rich, and detoxification system-friendly dish! This Basic Homemade Pumpkin Seed Butter recipe by Nikki Stokes only has one ingredient: pumpkin seed products. Simply toss in a meal processor, get those little morsels creamed upward, and enjoy!

This Homemade pumpkin seed butter is buttery; it tastes almost the same as peanut butter (only better). It's also completely nut-free, making it ideal for allergy-friendly occasions. Oh yes, and it's a brilliant natural! Homemade pumpkin seed butter is super easy to make and contains only 1 ingredient - pumpkin seed products (also called pepitas). Use it just as you would make use of all of your preferred nut butter--on sandwiches, with celery sticks, or in sweets. You'll be amazed at how tasty it is!

Calories 108

Serves 25

Cooking Time 30

Ingredients

3 cups of pumpkin seed products/pepitas

Preparation

- Process until clean, stopping at normal intervals to be sure the pumpkins seed butter doesn't overheat.
- Store inside jars in the fridge. Helps to keep for weeks.

Notes

Making pumpkin seed butter - or any nut or seed butter - can be hard on your food processor. In case your motor feels as though it's getting scorching while milling your pumpkin seed products, turn it off and keep it for at least

30 minutes to allow the motor to cool off. You can even rest at intervals (five minutes) through the process, to help keep temperatures down.

Seaweed and Tofu Poke

Seaweed is a superb plant-based food your detoxifying diet will like! This Seaweed and Tofu Poke recipe by Molly Patrick consists of wakame, which is "extremely nutrient-dense; provides higher amounts of metal, omega-3's, supplement A, proteins, magnesium, B nutritional vitamins, iodine, and chlorophyll." You're dousing the body with everything good!

Poke is a traditional Hawaiian meal made from Ahi Tuna. This poke uses tofu and seaweed tossed in ginger, lime, garlic clove, onions, and soy sauce. Wakame, which is a kind of kelp, can be included in the meal. Love this particular seafood-inspired meal nice and chilly.

Ingredients

14-ounce package additional firm tofu, cut into bite-sized

cubes

2 tablespoons dried wakame, soaked in water for at least 10 minutes

3 tablespoons soy sauce

2 tablespoons sesame seeds

2 teaspoons lime juice

2 garlic clove cloves, minced

1/2 cup red onion, finely diced

1/2 teaspoon ginger, peeled and grated

2 natural onions, chopped

Preparation

- Place the dried wakame inside a medium-sized dish and cover it with two glasses of water. Set this aside for a while, or prepare it, with regards to the instructions in the package.
- Wash the tofu with water and then draw out as much water as you possibly can by placing it in a pie skillet and stacking some plates together with it. Allow it to sit this way for 20 minutes while you prepare the other ingredients.

- In a big mixing bowl, add the soy sauce, sesame seeds, lime juice, garlic, red onion, ginger, and red onions.

- Remove the tofu from the pie pan, reduce into bite-sized cubes, and enhance the mixing bowl.

- Drain water from your seaweed, wash it with water and squeeze out as much water from it as possible. Add it in the mixing bowl with the tofu.

- Softly stir until all the ingredients are combined. Eat immediately or chill in the fridge. Serve cold.

Chia Burger Buns

Aside from sunflower, pumpkin, and hemp, chia seed products are also good foods to aid your lymphatic system. This Chia Burger Buns recipe by Aurora Steen is not only good for your lymph circulation, but it's also a super healthy and tasty choice for all those gluten-free people in the market who would still like the fulfilling fluff of a good burger bun!

These chia burger buns have the fluffy consistency you want in a burger bun and are a lot healthier! They're made from buckwheat flour and millet flakes, and also have the benefits of flax and chia seed products.

Ingredients

2 tablespoons chia seeds

1 cup of water

1 cup buckwheat flour

1 cup millet flakes

1 cup ground flaxseeds

1 tablespoon psyllium husk powder

3 teaspoons cooking powder

1/2 teaspoon salt

1 cup of water

2 tablespoons oil

Preparation

- Add all the ingredients in a dish and allow it to settle for 20 mins.
- Roll out 6 buns of the same size and place them on the baking holder with parchment papers.
- At 390°F, bake the buns for 45 a few minutes.

Fizzy Red Grapefruit Lemonade

Grapefruit might be a bitter fruit to swallow for a few, nonetheless it "contains two main antioxidants: naringin and naringenin" which help to "protect the liver from injuries by reducing swelling and protecting the liver cells." Also, these same substances "can also decrease fat buildup in the liver and increase the enzymes that get rid of fat." This Fizzy Green Grapefruit Lemonade recipe by Melissa Tedesco has only three easy components: grapefruit, maple syrup, and water. Super basic, yummy, and liver boosting!

Ingredients

2 pink grapefruits

2 tablespoons maple syrup (or even more if you want it sweeter)

1-liter soda drinking water (or any clean water)

lime wedges for garnish (optional)

Preparation

- Peel every of the pores and skin and pith (whitened part) from the grapefruits and reduce them into pieces.

- Blend the grapefruit and maple syrup in a blender until it's clean.
- Pour the blended grapefruit by way of a sieve right into a jug.
- Add the soft drinks or clean drinking water.
- Serve chilled or higher ice with a lime garnish.